AF787312

Healthcare Access - Regional Overviews

Edited by Umar Bacha,
Urška Rozman and Sonja Šostar Turk

Published in London, United Kingdom

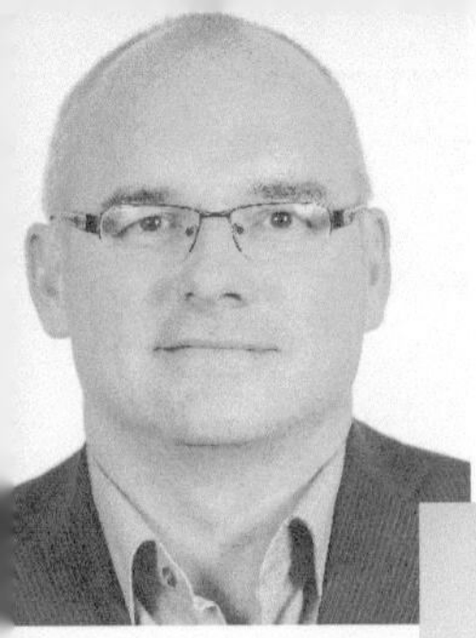
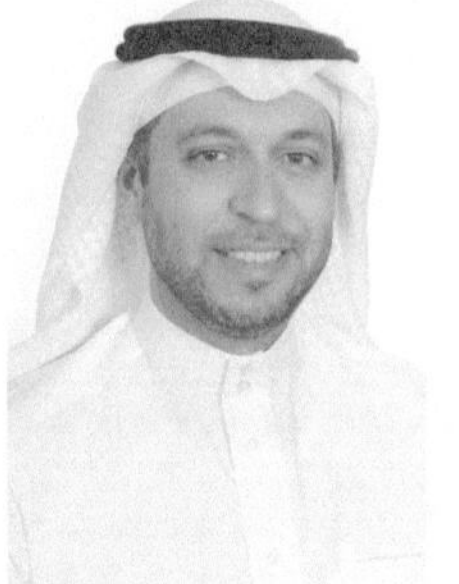
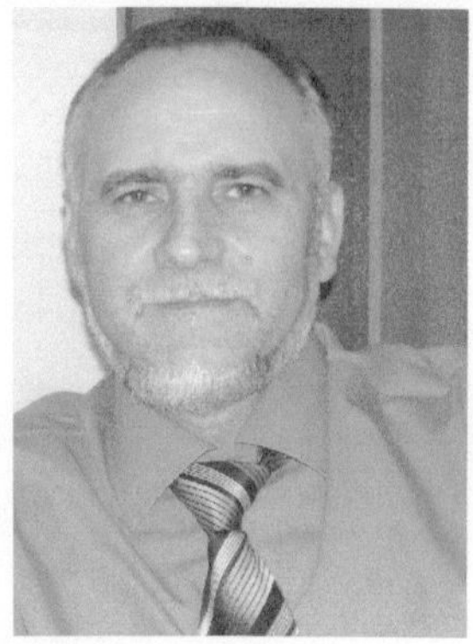
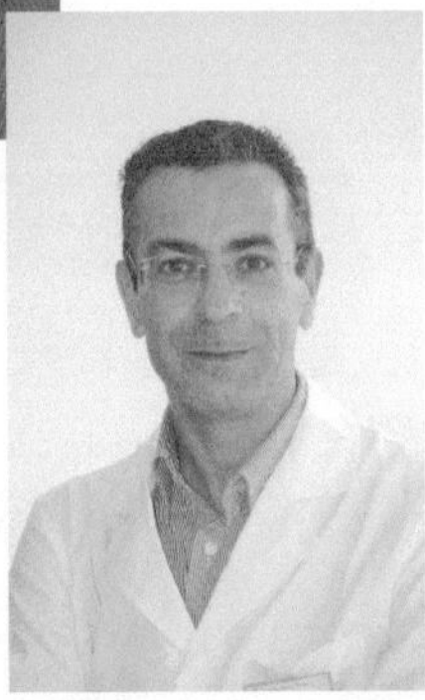
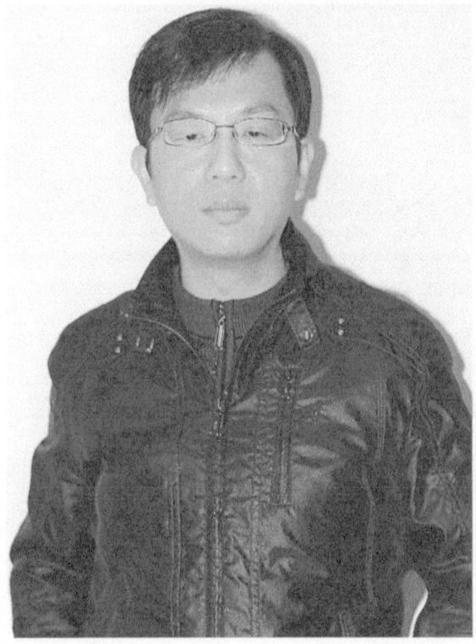
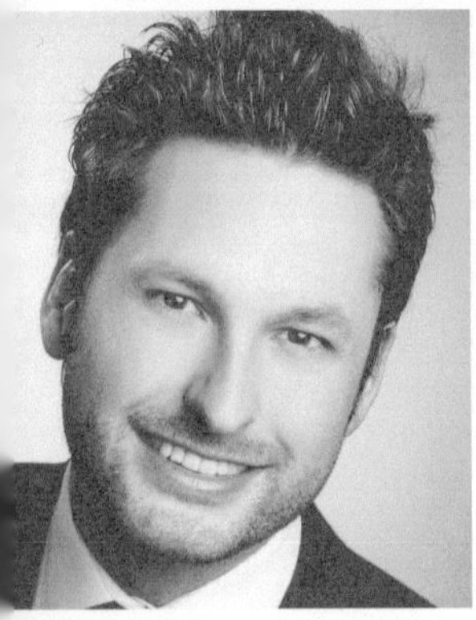
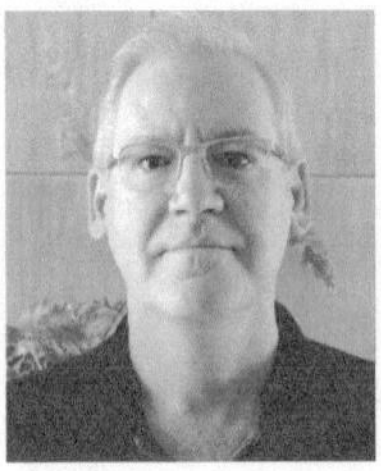

IntechOpen

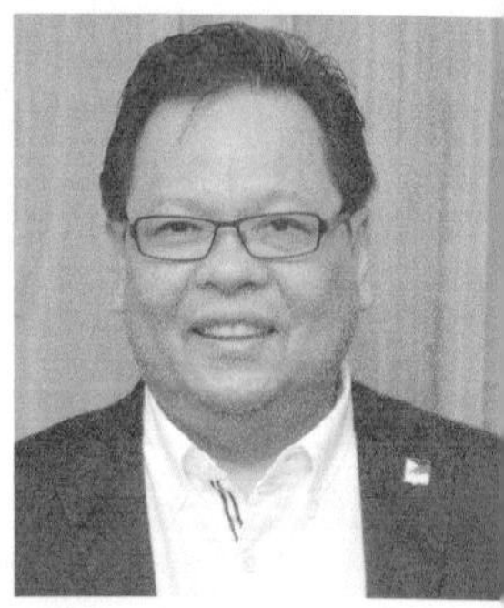
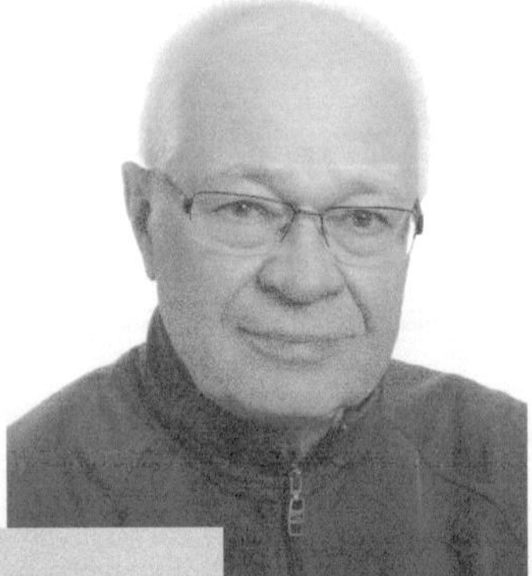
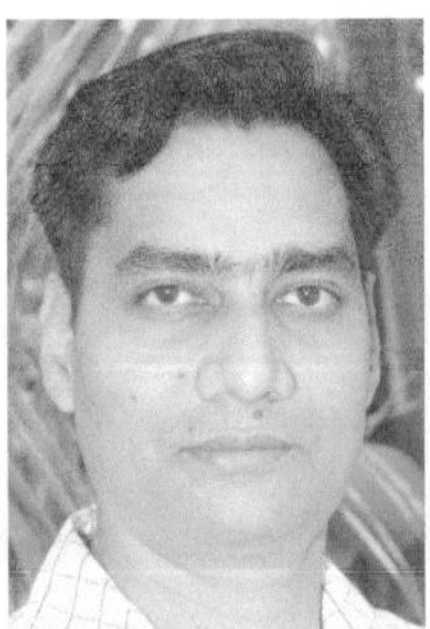
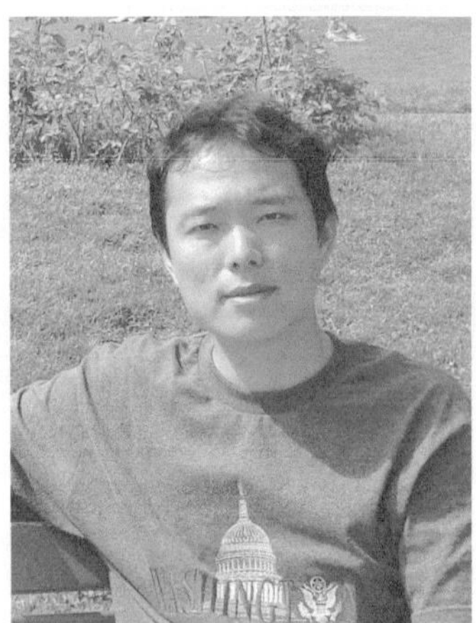
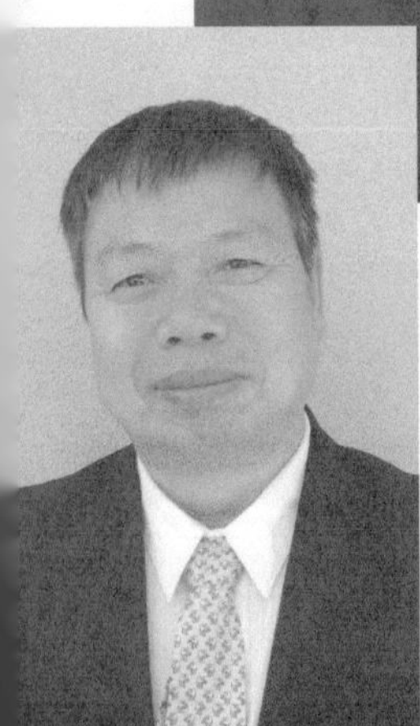
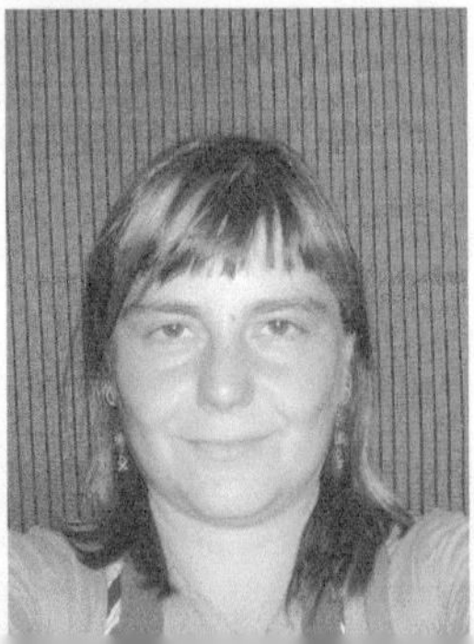

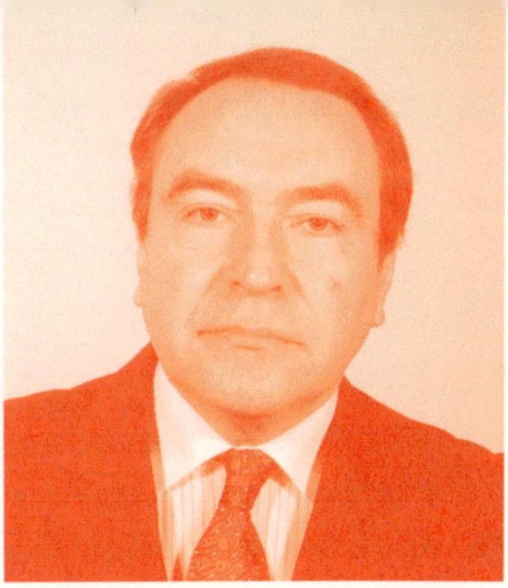
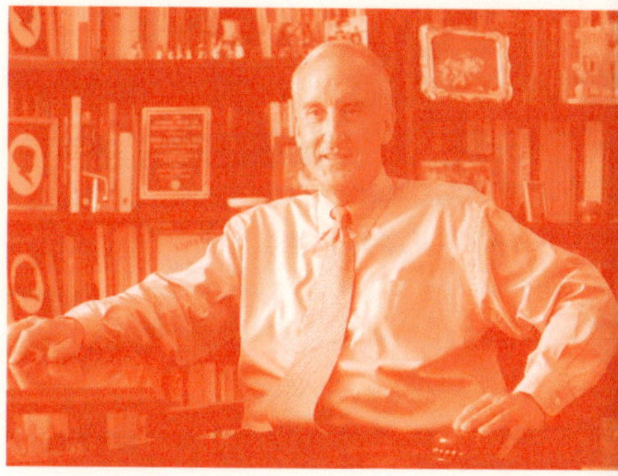
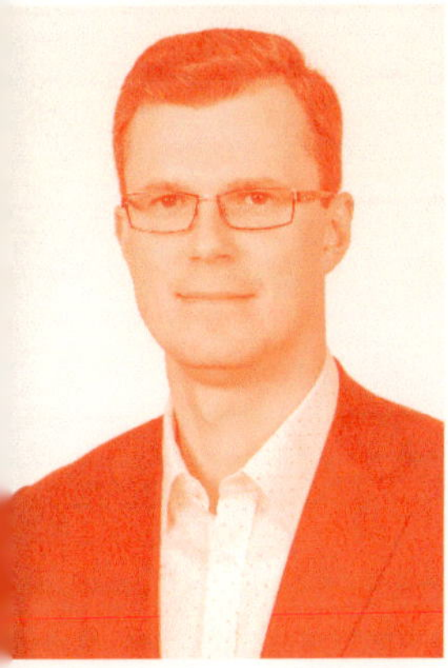
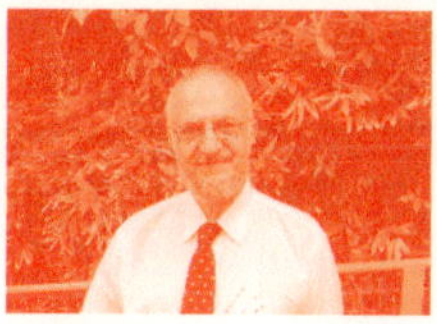
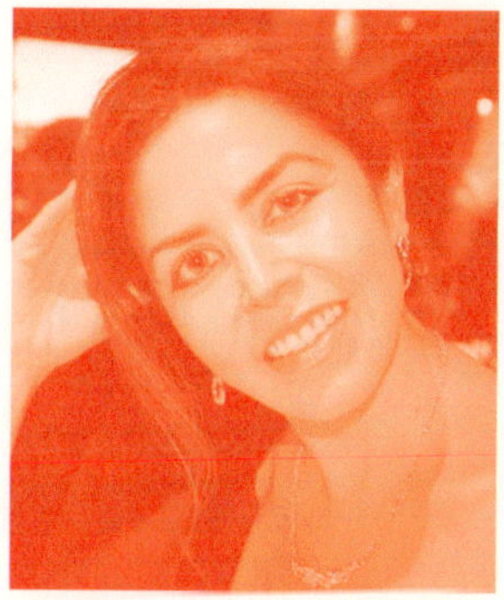

Supporting open minds since 2005

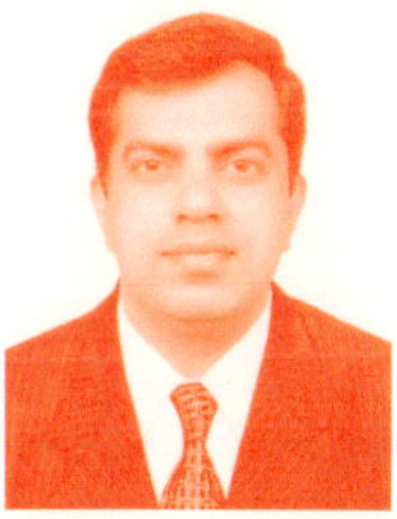
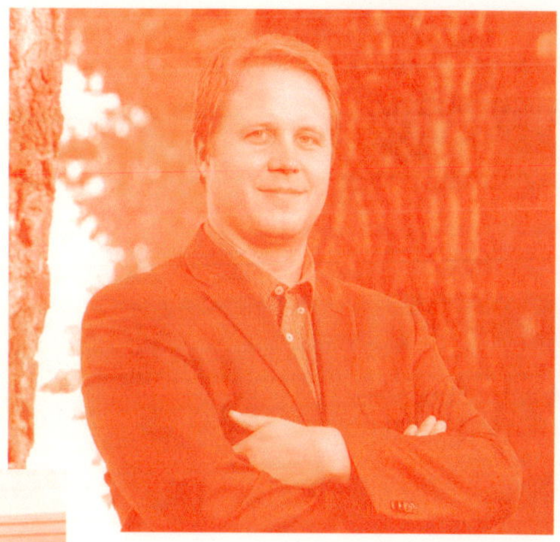
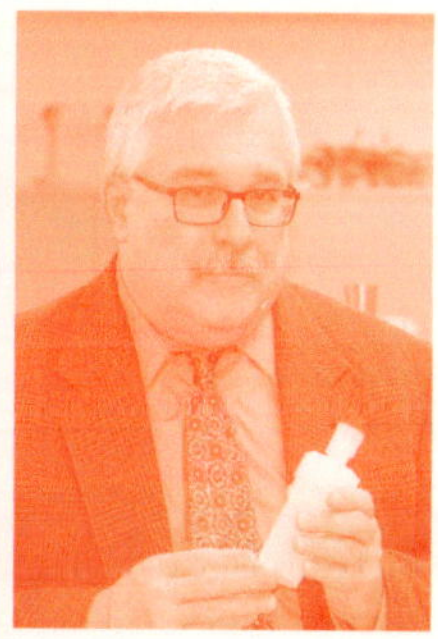
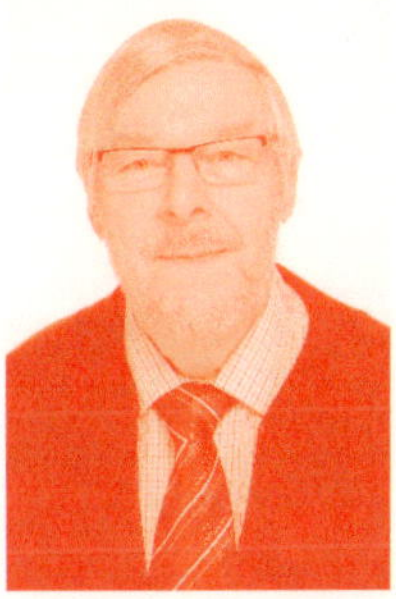
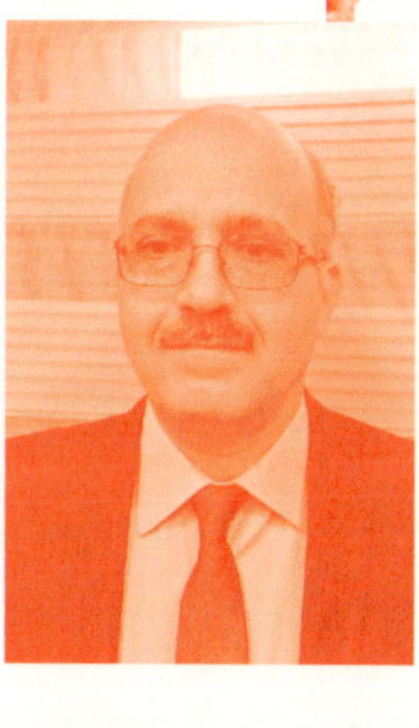
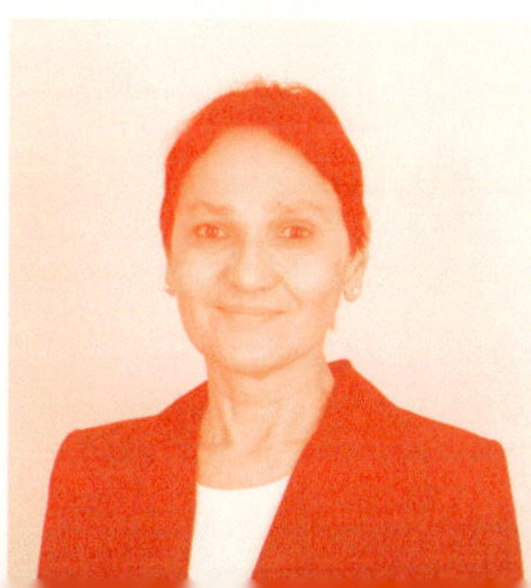
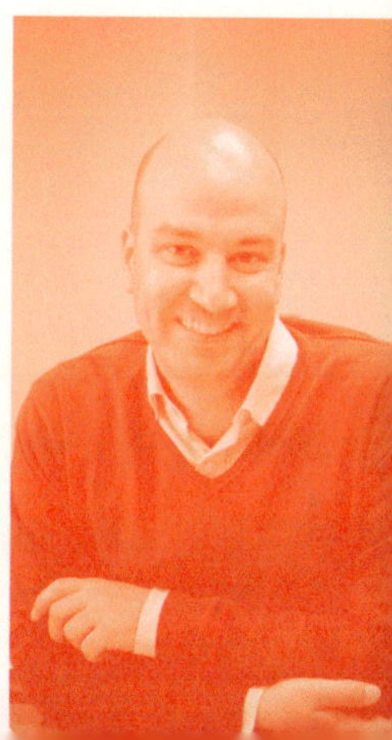

Healthcare Access - Regional Overviews
http://dx.doi.org/10.5772/intechopen.77867
Edited by Umar Bacha, Urška Rozman and Sonja Šostar Turk

Contributors
Muhammad Danasabe Isah, Muhammad Aliyu Makusidi, Kyaw San Lin, Andrew W Taylor-Robinson, Karen Bullock, Ramona Bullock-Johnson, Asimina Kaiafa Saropoulou, Stavros Yannopoulos, Abdul-Moomin Adams, Ibrahim Abu Abdulai, Juliet Waterkeyn, Sandy Cairncross, Amans Ntakarutimana, Anthony Waterkeyn, Julia Pantoglou, Regis Matimati, Joseph Katabarwa, Andrew Muringniza, Agrippa Chingono, Zachary Bigirimana, Edgar Cambaza, Edson Mongo, Robina Nhambire, Elda Anapakala, Jacinto Singo, Edsone Machava, Peter O Otieno, Gershim Asiki, Teodora Larisa Timis, Daniela-Rodica Mitrea, Ioan Alexandru Florian

© The Editor(s) and the Author(s) 2020
The rights of the editor(s) and the author(s) have been asserted in accordance with the Copyright, Designs and Patents Act 1988. All rights to the book as a whole are reserved by INTECHOPEN LIMITED. The book as a whole (compilation) cannot be reproduced, distributed or used for commercial or non-commercial purposes without INTECHOPEN LIMITED's written permission. Enquiries concerning the use of the book should be directed to INTECHOPEN LIMITED rights and permissions department (permissions@intechopen.com).
Violations are liable to prosecution under the governing Copyright Law.

CC BY

Individual chapters of this publication are distributed under the terms of the Creative Commons Attribution 3.0 Unported License which permits commercial use, distribution and reproduction of the individual chapters, provided the original author(s) and source publication are appropriately acknowledged. If so indicated, certain images may not be included under the Creative Commons license. In such cases users will need to obtain permission from the license holder to reproduce the material. More details and guidelines concerning content reuse and adaptation can be found at http://www.intechopen.com/copyright-policy.html.

Notice
Statements and opinions expressed in the chapters are these of the individual contributors and not necessarily those of the editors or publisher. No responsibility is accepted for the accuracy of information contained in the published chapters. The publisher assumes no responsibility for any damage or injury to persons or property arising out of the use of any materials, instructions, methods or ideas contained in the book.

First published in London, United Kingdom, 2020 by IntechOpen
IntechOpen is the global imprint of INTECHOPEN LIMITED, registered in England and Wales, registration number: 11086078, 7th floor, 10 Lower Thames Street, London, EC3R 6AF, United Kingdom
Printed in Croatia

British Library Cataloguing-in-Publication Data
A catalogue record for this book is available from the British Library

Additional hard and PDF copies can be obtained from orders@intechopen.com

Healthcare Access - Regional Overviews
Edited by Umar Bacha, Urška Rozman and Sonja Šostar Turk
p. cm.
Print ISBN 978-1-83880-131-1
Online ISBN 978-1-83880-132-8
eBook (PDF) ISBN 978-1-83880-772-6

For EU product safety concerns:
IN TECH d.o.o., Prolaz Marije Krucifikse Kozulić 3, 51000 Rijeka, Croatia, info@intechopen.com or visit our website at intechopen.com.

We are IntechOpen, the world's leading publisher of Open Access books

Built by scientists, for scientists

4,800+
Open access books available

123,000+
International authors and editors

135M+
Downloads

151
Countries delivered to

Our authors are among the
Top 1%
most cited scientists

12.2%
Contributors from top 500 universities

WEB OF SCIENCE™

Selection of our books indexed in the Book Citation Index in Web of Science™ Core Collection (BKCI)

Interested in publishing with us?
Contact book.department@intechopen.com

Numbers displayed above are based on latest data collected.
For more information visit www.intechopen.com

Meet the editors

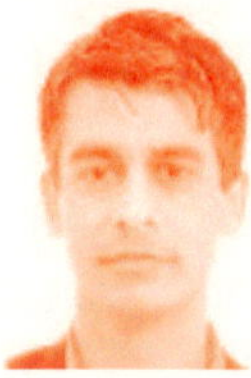

Umar Bacha, PhD, is Assistant Professor at the School of Health Sciences, University of Management and Technology, Lahore, Pakistan while also serving as chairman of the department since 2019. He obtained a BSc Hon in Biochemistry and PhD in Nutrition. He has published several research papers and authored and coauthored several books. His field of interest includes nutrient and drug interactions with an emphasis on drugs' effect on nutrient bioavailability and public health nutrition. He has several national and international awards to his credit.

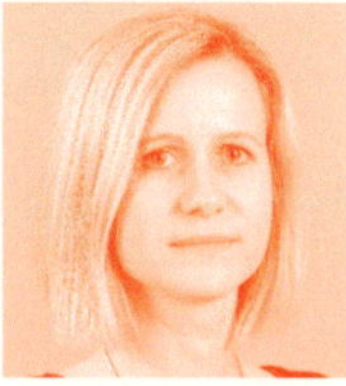

Urška Rozman is Assistant Professor of Biology at the Faculty of Health Sciences, University of Maribor, Maribor, Slovenia. Dr. Rozman has a university degree in Biology and Chemistry and a master's in Biology. She obtained a PhD in Ecology from the Faculty of Natural Sciences and Mathematics, University of Maribor, with study on molecular methods in microbiology for purposes of hospital hygiene. She participates in study programmes of Nursing, Bioinformatics, and Food Safety covering environmental factors affecting human health. She has participated in several research projects focusing on environmental microbiology, hospital and waste water hygiene, and nutrition.

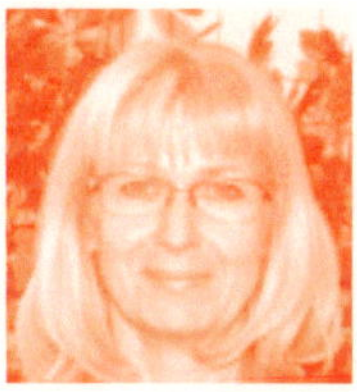

Sonja Šostar Turk, PhD, is Full Professor in the Faculty of Health Sciences, University of Maribor, Maribor, Slovenia, working in the research areas of textile chemistry, environmental engineering, and hygiene. She is the author of more than eighty original scientific papers, and has published around 250 scientific conference contributions. She was also involved in seventy-five national and international projects; most notably ten EU projects. She carried out preliminary studies for industry and health institutions. She is participating in study programmes of Nursing, Bioinformatics, and Food Safety covering subjects in the field of environmental factors affecting human health and hygiene. She has also participated in several research projects focusing on environmental health, hospital and waste water hygiene, and nutrition.

Contents

Preface

Healthcare Access - Regional Overviews and Reforms is a compilation of case studies, research works, reviews, and expert opinions providing insight on previous and current developments in the field of hygiene and infection control with practices to prevent or minimize the spread of infectious diseases. The book also addresses the status and healthcare access of the most neglected segments in less developed countries. All chapters are written by global researchers and edited by experts in the field. Readers will hopefully gain a deep understanding of the cutting-edge work and efforts being made in healthcare. The academic editors are thankful to all authors who have included their work in this book.

Dr. Umar Bacha
School of Health Sciences,
University of Management and Technology,
Lahore, Pakistan

Urška Rozman and Sonja Šostar Turk
Faculty of Health Sciences,
University of Maribor,
Maribor, Slovenia

Section 1

Healthcare Coverage and Sector Reforms

Chapter 1

Making Universal Health Coverage Effective in Low- and Middle-Income Countries: A Blueprint for Health Sector Reforms

Peter O. Otieno and Gershim Asiki

Abstract

Health sector reforms not only require attention to specific components but also a supportive environment. In low- and middle-income countries (LMICs), there is still much to be done on ensuring that people receive prioritized healthcare services. Despite LIMCs spending an average of 6% of their GDP on health, there have been minimal impacts compared to high-income countries. Health sector reform is a gradual process with complex systems; hence, the need for a vision and long-term strategies to realize the desired goals. In this chapter, we present our proposal to advance universal health coverage (UHC) in LMICs. Overall, our main aim is to provide strategies for achieving actual UHC and not aspirational UHC in LMICs by strengthening health systems, improving health insurance coverage and financial protection, and reducing disparities in healthcare coverage especially on prioritized health problems, and enhancing a primary care-oriented healthcare system.

Keywords: universal health coverage, health sector reform, health systems, low- and middle-income countries

1. Introduction

More than three-quarters of the world's population now live in low- and middle-income countries with the largest burden of infectious and non-communicable diseases [1]. Unlike the developed countries, LMICs are characterized by inadequate resources and lack of pragmatic interventions to tackle this crippling yet increasing disease burden [2]. Demographic and epidemiological transitions are fast shifting the disease burden from communicable to NCDs with LMICs contributing to more than two-thirds of the global burden of NCDs [3]. The preparedness of most LMICs to respond to these changes is questionable, with most countries still grappling with inequities in access to healthcare resulting from the pluralistic and fragmented healthcare systems [2]. As a result, most LMICs countries are currently undergoing profound health sector reforms as strongly influenced by international bodies such as the World Health Organization (WHO), World Bank,

IntechOpen

the Inter-American Development Bank, and the International Monetary Fund. While some of the reform objectives are specific to each country, a common central focus has been around the need to develop a robust mechanism that ensures an efficient allocation of scarce resources and equitable healthcare access based on population needs.

Most of the LMICs have set universal health coverage (UHC) as an aspirational goal for national health sector reform [4]. The dimensions of UHC as envisaged by the World Health Organization comprises of three key elements: the proportion of the national population that is covered by pooled funds; the proportion of direct healthcare costs covered by pooled funds; and the health services covered by those funds [4]. Reich et al. classified four distinct groups of LMICs at different points along the UHC ladder: The first group comprises countries such as Bangladesh and Ethiopia found at the bottom of the UHC ladder. The countries in this group are still grappling with the integration of the UHC agenda within the national policy. The second group comprises countries such as Indonesia, Peru, and Vietnam that have made significant progress toward UHC but still face huge gaps in coverage. The third group comprises of countries, such as Brazil, Thailand, and Turkey that have attained several UHC policy goals but are still struggling with the sustainability issues. The fourth group comprises countries such as France and Japan that have already achieved UHC but still need to implement major national policy adjustments targeting demographic and epidemiological challenges of aging populations and the increasing prevalence of degenerative diseases as well as innovations in technology [5].

In this chapter, we develop our proposals to advance UHC in LMICs. The chapter includes an overview of the health system in LMIC, the driving forces for changes, and our action plans to implement health sector reform for moving forward the UHC agenda in LMICs.

2. The healthcare system of LMICs

The healthcare systems of LMICs are highly fragmented across the public and private sector with expenditures averaging to 6% of GDP [6]. A recent report by the WHO has drawn attention to the weaknesses of the healthcare systems of LMICs. Of the 75 countries that account for more than 95% of maternal and child deaths, the median proportion of skilled birth attendance is only 62%, with pregnant mothers without financial protection at the highest risk of unskilled delivery [7]. **Figure 1** shows the health care financing sources according to a country's income. About half of health care financing in low-income countries comes from out-of-pocket payments, as compared to a third and in middle and a quarter high-income countries [8]. Thus, the financial protection of households from the already impoverishing effects of catastrophic health expenditures has been a major challenge for LMICs with only about a third of healthcare financing combined in funding pools [8].

Health insurance is considered by most LMIC as a promising means of achieving UHC [9]. Most countries have introduced various types of health insurance schemes with the commonest being National or social health insurance (SHI) which is based on mandatory insurance for formal sector employees [10]. Others include voluntary health insurance such as private health insurance (PHI) and community-based health insurance (CBI). The PHI have been implemented on a large scale in middle-income countries compared to low-income countries while CBHI are available in countries like Democratic republic of Congo, Ghana, Rwanda, and Senegal. [10]. The various types of health insurance may confer

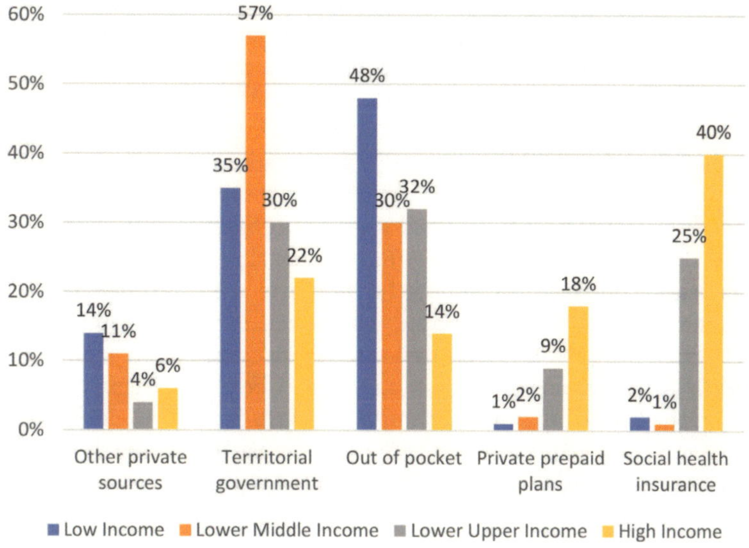

Figure 1.
Sources of healthcare financing.

different health impacts on the populations covered. For example, PHI mainly covers the affluent segments of a population while community-based health insurance (CBHI) is often preferred for the poor and the most vulnerable segment of the population [11]. Therefore, LMIC countries wishing to introduce health insurance schemes into their health systems must take into account the differences in various types of health insurance schemes. Studies on the population health by impacts of health insurance schemes in LMIC are scarce. Previous studies have evaluated the impacts of health insurance based on enrollment, financial management, and sustainability [2, 5, 12, 13]. A recent study on the performance of CBHI in LMICs, with a particular focus on China, Ghana, India, Mali, Rwanda, and Senegal revealed that the picture in Africa and Asia is very patchy [14]. Furthermore, the design of CBHI is heterogeneous with wide variations in population coverage, healthcare services covered and costs achieved [10]. The paucity of literature on the impact of SHI and PHI has resulted in a limited direct comparison of their options. Furthermore, most studies available on reforms in health insurance in LMIC are somewhat outdated.

The commitment by LMICs toward financial protection has been affirmed as part of the UHC. For example, countries in South and Southeast Asia such as the Philippines and Vietnam, have resorted to expand health insurance coverage by encouraging voluntary enrollment in social health insurance programs, while other countries, such as Thailand, have channeled funds from general taxation to the ministry of health and local authorities [15]. A recent report from the High-Level Expert Group on Universal Health Coverage in India recommended more financial allocations from the tax revenue base to public providers through a public purchaser at the state level as opposed to contributory insurance arrangements [16].

In Africa, Rwanda and Ghana have emerged as one of the countries with the highest health insurance coverage although the depth of the coverage is limited and there still exist financial protection gaps between the rich and the poor in both countries [13, 17]. The national health insurance program in Ghana is compulsory for every individual in the formal sector and voluntary for those in the informal sector and free for the poorest members of the population. However, the challenges of having affordable premiums and maintaining voluntary enrolment have prompted the national government to propose a one-time payment rather than annual payment from those in the informal sector [13]. Given that the national healthcare system of Ghana is mainly financed by general taxation through value-added tax therefore the proposal to introduce a one-time payment would signal a decline in the importance attached to contributory insurance [13].

In view of the limited resources and narrow tax base, budgetary allocations in most LMICs to the healthcare sector have fallen short of the 15% envisaged in the Abuja declaration [18]. Consequently, there has been a limited ability of many households to pay for health care, whether directly or through health insurance. While progress toward universal health coverage may inevitably be gradual, LMIC countries need to draw on a mix of healthcare financing sources. In particular, the financing options should take into account the diversities in the economic, social, and political environment and ensure that the most vulnerable segment of the population is financially protected with a reasonable depth of coverage.

2.1 Driving forces for changes

Despite LIMCs spending an average of 6% of its GDP on health, there have been minimal impacts compared to high-income countries. The health care system challenges in LMICs can be observed throughout the public and private sectors. First, public health services delivery is highly fragmented, and implementation of decentralization policies has failed in most LMICs. Also, there is a lack of primary care orientation, low institutional capacity, poor health information systems, and widespread inequalities in health care utilization. Second, most LMICs have low health insurance coverage and limited financial protection of households from the impoverishing effects of catastrophic health expenditures mainly due to the high levels of unemployment and poor management of pooled resources via the national health insurance schemes.

In the private health sector, problems arise due to a rigid regulatory framework that has resulted in the proliferation of private health providers which are unregulated, unaccountable, and out of control. In most LMICs, the growth of the private health sector has been characterized by poor planning and government reluctance in monitoring licensing provisions. Most health professional councils are defunct and being misused by the dominant vested interests. Although equity in health service delivery and availability of health resources including human power have featured in policy documents of LMICs, the legal and licensing provisions for healthcare providers, setting up health facilities are not often seriously enforced. As a result, there is gross imbalance between the actual growth of the physical services and the quality of healthcare services provided.

3. A blueprint for health sector reforms in LMICs

To achieve effective UHC, meaning that people receive quality prioritized healthcare services resulting in the actual translation of goals into out-come improvements on prioritized conditions, the LMIC countries will need to address and correct some of the dysfunctional gears in the health system. In approaching this health sector reform process, we have decided to focus on several key issues (see **Table 1**). After describing each strategic challenge, we provide our proposed actions for reform. This is our blueprint for health sector reforms in LMICs.

Key issue	Strategy
Community and household level	
• Physical, social, and financial barriers to access	• Focus on expanding "close to client services," for example, primary care services provided by community health volunteers (CHVs) • Improve financial protection by expanding health insurance coverage and removing financial barriers at the point of use • Improve responsiveness of the health service delivery through pay for performance approaches
• Poor demand for evidence-based interventions	• Community mobilization by creation of support groups and welfare organizations to spread health information such as antenatal care and screening for chronic illnesses
Healthcare service delivery	
• Inadequate qualified health workforce especially at primary care level	• Increase number of qualified staff • Implement task shifting by training CHVs to treat common illness • Increase allowance for work in remote areas
• Lack of motivation of staff and low remuneration, weak technical guidance, program management, and supervision	• Increase salaries sustainably and strengthen training and support supervision
• Inadequate medical supplies and equipment, poor health infrastructure, and limited access to healthcare services	• Improve public supply systems and utilize private retail system • Allocate adequate resources for renovating, upgrading, and expanding public facilities, contract nongovernmental organizations to provide services
Policy and strategy management in health sector	
• Fragmented and overly centralized planning and management systems	• Decentralize planning and management
• Weak drug policies and supplies system	• Introduce new supply mechanisms
• Rigid regulatory frameworks and proliferation unregulated, unaccountable, and out of control private health sector	• Strengthen regulation through enforcement legal mechanisms, for example, licensing provisions for healthcare providers and setting up health facilities
• Poor cooperative action and partnership between civic organizations and government	• Engagement of civic organizations in planning and service oversight
• Weak incentives to use inputs efficiently and to respond to user needs and preferences	• Use of output-based payments and external assistance programs
• Fragmented donor funding, which reduces flexibility and ownership; low priority given to systems support	• Implement reforms to aid management and delivery (e.g., sector wide approaches and International Health Partnership Plus) • Provide increased financing for systems support
Political and physical environment	
• Governance and overall policy framework (e.g., corruption, weak government, weak rule of law and enforceability of contracts, political instability and insecurity, social sectors not given priority in funding decisions, and weak structure for public accountability)	• Encourage improved stewardship and accountability mechanisms by encouraging growth in civic organizations

Key issue	Strategy
Global health	
• Fragmented governance and management structures for global health	• Improve global coordination (e.g., the Paris Declaration, Accra Agenda for Action)
• Emigration of doctors and nurses to high-income countries	• Seek voluntary agreements on migration of doctors and nurses

Table 1.
Key issues faced by healthcare systems in LMICs and proposed action for reform.

4. Measuring and monitoring implementation

The essential components of the health sector reforms proposed in **Table 1** are only the gears to drive health sector reforms in LMICs to improve health outcomes. The realized gains from these reforms should be equitable distributed between and with LMICs. Monitoring progress of health sector reforms requires a robust health management information system embedded in a national interoperability plan. The measurable standards at the national at global level can be obtained level can be obtained from this plan to ensure that information generated can be harmonized and used for surveillance, monitoring, and evaluation of interventions and policies and clinical decision making at the point of care.

Enhancing prevention, promotion, treatment, rehabilitation, and palliative care to people in need without financial hardship as envisaged in the UHC requires major focus on the three interrelated components of UHC: first, ensuring a full spectrum of quality health services according to the needs; second, improving financial protection from direct payment for health services when consumed; and, lastly, expanding coverage for the entire population. In this regard, we propose a system of UHC monitoring in LMICs that will ensure that progress toward UHC reflects the unique epidemiological and demographic profiles of LMICs as well as the population demands and levels of economic development. The monitoring and evaluation plan for UHC in LMIC should include two guiding principles: financial protection and coverage of healthcare services. The primary outcomes include effectiveness, equity, and quality of healthcare at all levels of the health system for the full population across the life cycle, including all ages and genders.

5. Conclusions

Health sector reforms in LMIC not only require a central focus on the health systems components but also a supportive environment for innovation and change. Health sector reform is a gradual process with complex systems hence the need for a vision and long-term strategies to realize the desired goals. Although most LMICs have prioritized UHC in their national policy agenda, there are still needs to work on achieving effective UHC, especially with regard to quality and equity. Therefore, the LMIC should focus on achieving actual and not aspirational UHC by strengthening health systems by improving health insurance coverage and financial protection, improving access to healthcare, reducing disparities in healthcare coverage especially on prioritized health problems, and enhancing a primary care-oriented healthcare system.

Conflict of interest

The authors declare no conflict of interest.

Author details

Peter O. Otieno* and Gershim Asiki
African Population and Health Research Center, Nairobi, Kenya

*Address all correspondence to: pootienoh@gmail.com

IntechOpen

© 2020 The Author(s). Licensee IntechOpen. This chapter is distributed under the terms of the Creative Commons Attribution License (http://creativecommons.org/licenses/by/3.0), which permits unrestricted use, distribution, and reproduction in any medium, provided the original work is properly cited.

References

[1] Wang H et al. GBD 2015 mortality and causes of death collaborators. Global, regional, and national life expectancy, all-cause mortality, and cause-specific mortality for 249 causes of death, 1980-2015: A systematic analysis for the global burden of disease study 2015. The Lancet. 2016;**388**(10053):1459-1544

[2] Bollyky TJ et al. Lower-income countries that face the most rapid shift in noncommunicable disease burden are also the least prepared. Health Affairs. 2017;**36**(11):1866-1875

[3] Daniels M, Donilon T, Bollyky TJ. The Emerging Global Health Crisis: Noncommunicable Diseases in Low-and Middle-Income Countries. Council on Foreign Relations Independent Task Force Report No. 72; 2014

[4] World health organization (WHO). The World Health Report 2010: Health Systems Financing: The Path to Universal Coverage. World health organization (WHO); 2010

[5] Reich MR et al. Moving towards universal health coverage: Lessons from 11 country studies. The Lancet. 2016;**387**(10020):811-816

[6] World Bank. Financing Health in Middle-Income Countries; 2019

[7] World Health Organization and UNICEF. Countdown to 2015: Accountability for Maternal, Newborn and Child Survival: The 2013 Update. World Health Organization and UNICEF; 2013

[8] World Health Organization. Global Health Expenditure Database. Available from: http://apps.who.int/nha/database/CompositionReportPage.aspx

[9] WHO. The World Health Report 2010: Health Systems Financing: The Path to Universal Coverage. World Health Organization (WHO); 2010;**1**:2-3

[10] Spaan E et al. The impact of health insurance in Africa and Asia: A systematic review. Bulletin of the World Health Organization. 2012;**90**:685-692

[11] Smith KV, Sulzbach S. Community-based health insurance and access to maternal health services: Evidence from three west African countries. Social Science & Medicine. 2008;**66**(12):2460-2473

[12] Otieno PO et al. Prevalence and factors associated with health insurance coverage in resource-poor urban settings in Nairobi, Kenya: A cross-sectional study. BMJ Open. 2019;**9**(12):1-2

[13] Abiiro GA, McIntyre D. Universal financial protection through National Health Insurance: A stakeholder analysis of the proposed one-time premium payment policy in Ghana. Health Policy and Planning. 2012;**28**(3):263-278

[14] Soors W et al. Community Health Insurance and Universal Coverage: Multiple Paths, Many Rivers to Cross. World Health Organization; 2010

[15] Tangcharoensathien V et al. Health-financing reforms in Southeast Asia: Challenges in achieving universal coverage. The Lancet. 2011;**377**(9768):863-873

[16] High Level Expert Group. Report on Universal Health Coverage for India: Submitted to the Planning Commission of India. New Delhi; 2011. pp. 3-4

[17] Lu C et al. Towards universal health coverage: An evaluation of Rwanda Mutuelles in its first eight years. PLoS One. 2012;7(6):e39282

[18] WHO. The Abuja Declaration: Ten Years on; 2019

Chapter 2

Access to Maternal Healthcare Services under the National Health Insurance Policy in the Upper West Region, Ghana

Ibrahim Abu Abdulai and Abdul-Moomin Adams

Abstract

Health insurance coverage provides the spring board for pregnant women to access and utilise maternal healthcare services. Yet, studies on health insurance coverage, access and utilisation of maternal healthcare are a handful. Consequently, this study examines women's access and utilisation of maternal healthcare services under the free maternal health policy in two districts in northern Ghana. The study adopted the mixed research approach with the aid of the cross-sectional design involving 212 respondents. An interview schedule was utilised in the collection of data. Percentages, Chi-square test for independence and Mann-Whitney U test as well as thematic analysis were used to analyse the data. The study revealed that 93.9% of the respondents had enrolled unto the national health insurance scheme and 98.6% of them went for antennal care. Majority (66.5%) of them had facility-based delivery. However, 79.7% of them incur cost in seeking delivery care. In brief, health insurance coverage appears to contribute to improved access and utilisation of maternal healthcare services in the two districts. Nonetheless, the government should provide the basic items that are needed for delivery to lessen the cost burden associated with facility-based delivery.

Keywords: healthcare, health, insurance, maternal, Ghana

1. Introduction

Access to healthcare including maternal healthcare services drives public health policies across the globe [1–3]. According to Ribot [4], access connotes the ability to make use of a resource. In the field of maternal healthcare, access entails the ability of women to obtain prenatal, antenatal, facility-based delivery and postnatal services [5] since these services contribute to beneficial health outcome for both the baby, and mother. Hence, Krutilova [6] maintains that all individuals including women ought to have access to healthcare that meet their needs regardless of their economic, social and physical attributes. Yet, access to maternal healthcare services remains a major development challenge around the world and in Africa, the state of affairs is more disquieting [6]. In sub-Saharan Africa in particular, Twum et al. [7] posit that financial constraints tend to erect barriers to access healthcare for the less privileged, particularly women. As a result, Kibusi et al. [8] pointed out that

IntechOpen

maternal mortality ratio in Sub-Saharan Africa continues to rise despite the many interventions such as health insurance.

Health insurance, therefore, comes in handy as it provides a mechanism for pregnant women to access and utilise maternal healthcare services. Ho [9] elucidates that health insurance protects the poor in particular against the risk of incurring medical and related financial costs at the point of service utilisation. In addition, Dalinjong et al. [10] emphasise that health insurance coverage allows all pregnant women to access maternal health services throughout pregnancy, childbirth, and post-delivery. Further, health insurance plays a critical role in improving maternal mortality ratio and related health outcomes [8]. Thus, governments have the responsibility to capture all persons including women under a health insurance scheme [11] to protect them against incurring financial cost at the point of maternal health services utilisation as insinuated by the social justice theory.

The social justice theory's core arguments centre on fairness and equality. As such, all people have a right to fair treatment and an equal share of the benefits of society [12] including health insurance coverage and consequently access to maternal health services. Also, Jost and Kay [13] elucidate that social justice ensures that societal benefits and obligations are shared in accordance with acceptable procedures, norms and rules that promote basic rights, liberties and entitlement of individuals and or groups within a society. Furthermore, social justice involves a fair and equal access to primary goods such as maternal healthcare services [14]. Bankson [15] contributes that social justice encourages the redistribution of goods and resources such as maternal health services in a way that improves the situations of the disadvantaged. In a nutshell, social justice is predicated on equal access and in the view of Nussbaum [16], efforts should be geared towards removing the obstacles that perpetuate differences, marginalisation or discrimination based on geographical location. Thus, health insurance coverage appears to provide a window of opportunity to reduce Out-of-pocket expenditure [17] and ease access to maternal healthcare services.

Access theory is hinged on the ability of the individual/or group to benefits from resources such as health insurance through acceptable processes [4, 18]. Ribot and Peluso [18] conceive access to mean the ability of the individual/or group to benefit from such things as material objects, persons, institutions, and symbols. Therefore, the central tenets of access theory are maintenance, and control which are mediated by institutional structures and processes [4] within a social system. According to Ribot [4], maintenance concerns expending resources for individual/or collective benefit, whereas power over others constitutes control. In addition, Ribot and Peluso [18] intimate that power constitutes the material, cultural and political-economic constituents within the social setup that spell out access to resources such as maternal healthcare. In brief, the expending of national resources in the form of free enrolment of pregnant women onto the national health insurance scheme [NHIS] seeks to guarantee access and utilisation of maternal healthcare services.

According to the World Health Statistics [19], 303, 000 women died as a result of pregnancy related causes in 2015. WHO further notes that 99% of the deaths occurred in low and middle-income countries (LMIC) and 64% of these deaths occurred in Africa. Previously, WHO [20] had estimated that Sub-Saharan Africa alone accounted for about 66% of global maternal related deaths. Specifically, Nigeria and India accounted for 19% and 15% respectively of global maternal deaths in 2015 [20]. Therefore, it is imperative for governments to ensure that women have access to quality care before, during and after childbirth since this will improve maternal mortality ratio [19]. Suffice it to say, the level of maternal mortality may have stimulated the formulation of sustainable development goals (SDGs) since health is fundamentally linked to sustainable development. Specifically, goal 3 focuses on ensuring that all people including pregnant women enjoy healthy lives and wellbeing. Thus, governments are obliged to ensure the realisation of this important goal.

In 2003, Ghana introduced a NHIS as a measure to safeguard its population against out-pocket-payment at the point of accessing healthcare services [21] particularly maternal healthcare services. It is, however, important to note that the NHIS policy recognises that some sections of the society may not be able to make the minimum contribution to the scheme [22]. As a result, children under 18 years old, elderly above 70 years old, Social Security and National Insurance Trust (SSNIT) pensioners, pregnant women, and extreme poor do not pay the premium [22]. This signals that exemption of pregnant women from paying the premium seeks to do away with financial barriers to maternal healthcare services and thus, to reduce or eradicate pregnancy-related deaths.

However, in Ghana, a total of 955 women died from pregnancy related causes in 2016 [23]. Ghana Statistical Service (GSS), Ghana Health Service (GHS), and ICF [24] also report that pregnancy-related mortality ratio for Ghana hovers around 343 deaths per 100,000 live births. GHS [23] had earlier noted that Greater Accra recorded the highest number of maternal deaths and this can be attributed to the concentration of referral facilities in Accra. GHS adds that the Upper West Region accounted for only 2% of the total maternal deaths in Ghana [23]. Nevertheless, GHS [23] posits that the Upper West Region is characterised by scattered health facilities which contribute to poor access to healthcare. This begs the question of whether enrolment and exemption of pregnant women from the payment of the NHIS's premium guarantees access and utilisation of maternal healthcare service in the region.

The Wa West and Wa East districts are among the underprivileged in Ghana. In terms of health infrastructure and personnel, for instance, the Wa-West District is disadvantaged [25]. The District has one health centre and 27 community health planning services (CHPS) compounds that serve 81,348 people [25, 26] living in the 208 communities. The Wa East district also has its fair share of challenges. The district suffers from limited health facilities, insufficient health personnel, inaccessible communities, and poor road network [27]. This hints that perhaps the people and in particular pregnant women living in these districts may suffer deprivation and injustice as a result of the persistence of these challenges.

Still, studies that relate to access to maternal healthcare under Ghana's NHIS appear to ignore rural idiosyncrasies associated with access to maternal healthcare services. Using 2008 DHS data, Wang et al. [28] examine the impact of NHIS coverage on access to maternal healthcare services in Ghana and came to the conclusion that majority of pregnant women reported at least one antenatal care visit and facility-based delivery. The study presented a national picture but fell short of a discussion of access to maternal healthcare services in rural areas. In a related study, Twum et al. [7] investigated access to maternal healthcare services under NHIS's free maternal healthcare policy in relatively well-endowed urban towns of Kintampo and Jema. The authors reported that pregnant women who were covered under the free maternal healthcare policy completed the recommended four antenatal care visits and delivered in a health facility but did not go for postnatal care. Yet the study ignored rural anomalies, distance and waiting time at the facility as important ingredients of access to maternal healthcare.

This study contributes to knowledge, first, by shifting the fulcrum of analysis of access from property to maternal healthcare and secondly, it sheds light on how enrolment onto the NHIS contributes to access to maternal healthcare in the two rural districts in the Upper West Region. Therefore, the study seeks to address the following objectives: (1) assess how NHIS underwrites access to maternal healthcare services, and (2) examine the utilisation of maternal healthcare services under the NHIS policy. The paper is divided into six sections. The section following this discusses the concepts that underpin the study. Next, a review of some empirical studies that relate to the subject matter of the paper is presented. The fourth section presents the methodology adopted for the study and the fifth section presents the empirical evidence of the study, while conclusions and policy implications constitute the final section.

2. Conceptual discussions

WHO [29] describes maternal health as the wellbeing of women before, during pregnancy, at childbirth and post-delivery. Therefore, maternal healthcare is concerned with providing pregnancy-related services to women and teen-age girls [24, 29]. Accordingly, maternal healthcare services include antenatal care (ANC), delivery care, and postnatal care (PNC) [24]. ANC denotes the care provided by skilled health workers to pregnant women and adolescent girls to ensure the best health conditions for the mother and baby [30]. Also, WHO notes that the uptake of ANC services enables skilled health personnel to identify risk, prevent risk and manage pregnancy-related diseases as well as engage in health education and promotion among pregnant women. Rutaremwa et al. [5] add that ANC attendance appears to help reduce stillbirths and neonatal death. Lincetto et al. [31] had earlier recommended that four ANC visits at specific intervals enable care givers to make essential interventions during pregnancy and subsequently during delivery.

Delivery care means attention given to mother during labour and delivery to respond to problems that may arise during the process. The care provided to women and new-borns until discharge is crucial for their health after they leave the health facility [20]. Further, WHO [30] noted that delivery care reduces illness and death in mothers and their new-borns babies. PNC, on the other hand, involves the provision of a supportive environment in which a woman, her baby and the wider family can begin their new life together [32]. According to Charlotte et al. [33], PNC ensures continuity of care for mother and baby as well as help to support healthy behaviours. Thus, PNC contributes to the beneficial health outcome for the baby as well as the mother [5]. Timilsina and Dhakal [34] also note that PNC helps to assess the health status of mother and new-born so as to be able to institute a remedy to any defect and to formulate preventive measure that may become necessary. It is, however, important to state that access to maternal healthcare services plays a crucial role in the utilisation of these services.

Access to healthcare refers to the ability of a given individual or group to enter into a health care delivery facility [35] and utilise the available services. In other words, access to health care describes the relationship between need, provision and utilisation of health services [36]. Therefore, access to maternal healthcare entails the entry into and use of skilled services during pregnancy, delivery and post-delivery [37]. However, the costs associated with seeking maternal healthcare services may discourage pregnant women, particularly the poor, from receiving healthcare services promptly [38]. As such, in 2003, the NHIS was introduced in Ghana and subsequently, in 2008, a free maternal healthcare programme (FMHCP) was set in motion to alleviate the cost burden associated with seeking maternal healthcare [7]. As a result, pregnant women do not pay a premium for fresh registration or renewal of membership and processing fees [7].

3. Empirical review

So far, our discussion is centred on the concepts that underpin the study. This section considers some empirical studies that have been carried out on health insurance and access to maternal healthcare services. Kibusi et al. [8] sought to find out whether health insurance coverage enabled pregnant women to utilise maternal health services in Tanzania. The study revealed that a small percentage of the respondents were covered by health insurance. Further, the results showed that the timing of the first ANC visit was also low and few women completed the recommended ANC visits. Yet, the authors found that majority of the respondents delivered at health facilities under skilled attendants and concluded that health insurance coverage was associated with the recommended timing of the first ANC visit as well as increases the chances for facility-based delivery. In Bangladesh, Banik [38] had earlier found that majority of pregnant women had their nearest health centre within a one-kilometre distance but had to wait for about an hour before being seen by the nurses or doctors. Also, decisions about seeking maternal healthcare services made by both husband and wife were higher compared to those made by husband or wife alone [38].

In a related study, Twum et al. [7] assessed the effectiveness of a free maternal healthcare programme under the NHIS in Ghana. The social justice and access theory undergird the study. The authors discovered that health insurance status of respondent played an important function in the use of maternal healthcare services and women with health insurance coverage had a better opportunity to use antenatal care, deliver at the facility and postnatal care compared with those who are not registered. Similarly, Dalinjong et al. [10] assessed the implementation of the free maternal health policy in rural Northern Ghana using the qualitative approach. The study found that women still paid for drugs, supplies, laboratory services including ultrasound scans and transport as well as the purchase of other items for childbirth. They also reported that distance and time taken to reach the nearest facility were impediments to seeking maternal healthcare. The next section of the paper discusses the study locations, sampling, data collection methods and instruments as well as data analysis techniques deployed in the study.

4. Study methods

The study was conducted in Wa West and Wa East Districts in the Upper West Region. The Wa West District is home to 81,348 people with 50.5% being females and the rest being males with a Total Fertility Rate of 4.1. The district is entirely rural and is located in the western part of the Upper West Region. The district lies between longitudes 9°40′N and 10°10′N and latitudes 2°20′W and 2°50′W. The southern part of the district is bordered by Northern Region, Nadowli-Kaleo District to the north-west, Wa Municipal to the east and Burkina Faso to the west [25]. The District occupies nearly 1492.0 km^2 and its capital, Wechiau is about 15.0 km away from Wa the regional capital. On the other hand, the Wa East district lies between latitudes 9°55′N and 10°25′N and longitude 1°10′W and 2°5′W and covers a land area of about 4297.1 km^2. The district capital, Funsi is about 115 km away from Wa and shares boundaries with West Mamprusi, West Gonja and the Sissala East district to the northwest, southeast and north, respectively. The district host about 72,074 inhabitants and 50.5% of them are males while the rest are females with a Total Fertility Rate of 3.9 [39]. **Figure 1** shows the zonal centres selected for the study.

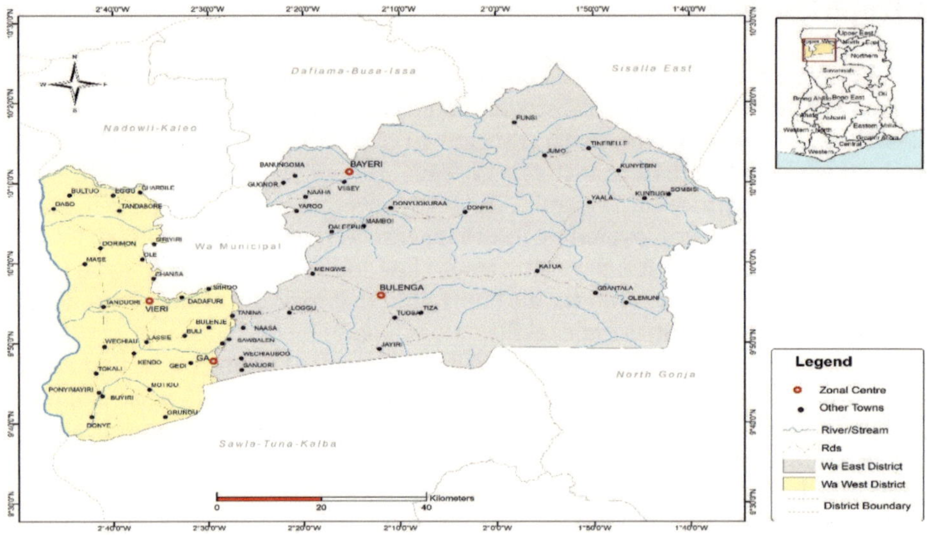

Figure 1.
Map of Wa East and Wa West show zonal centres sampled for the study. Source: adapted from GSS [25, 39].

The mixed research approach with the aid of the cross-sectional design which requires taking a snapshot of the phenomenon under consideration. However, the study was tilted towards the quantitative approach. The total number of households in the four sampled communities was 454. The sample size was computed using Yamane's statistical formula: $n = \frac{N}{1 + N(e)^2}$; where n is the sample size, N is the size of the study population, and e is the margin of error [40]. In this study, N = 454 and e = 0.05. The sample size was computed as: $n = \frac{454}{1 + 454(0.05)^2} = 212$. Therefore, the samples size for the study was 212 households.

The multi-stage sampling technique was deployed in selecting zonal centres, communities and households. First, Wa East district has four zonal centres: Funsi, Bulenga, Kulkpong, and Baayiri, whereas Ga, Gurungu, Vieri and Wechiau constitute the zonal centres for the Wa West District. Two zonal centres from each district (Bulenga, Baayiri, Vieri and Ga) (see **Figure 1**) were randomly selected to participate in the study. In each zonal centre, the names of the communities were compiled and one community was randomly selected. In all, four communities (Guonuo, Tampala, Ga, and Berenyasi) were randomly sampled for the study. Following on that one house was randomly selected and the subsequent houses were then systematically sampled after every fourth house. Finally, women within the reproductive ages of 15–49 years [41] who have had children between 2015 and 2019 were identified and interviewed. Interviewing was the method used to collect the data with the aid of an interview schedule which contained both open-ended and closed-ended questions. Descriptive statistics, chi-square test for independence, Man-Witney test and thematic analysis were deployed in the analysis of the data. The results were presented in tables, text and narration.

5. The evidence

5.1 Background characteristics of respondents

The results show that the maximum age of respondents was 42 years whereas the minimum age was 15 years with a median of 25 (Mean = 25.94; Std Deviation = 6.32;

Skewness = .749) with a quartile deviation of 4.5 years. This finding agrees with WHO [41] that reproductive age of women ranges between 15 and 49 years. The results also indicate that 93.9% of the respondents were married while the rest were single. As shown in **Table 1**, 48% of the respondents have no formal education whereas only 4.2% attained tertiary education. Also, 41% of them were engaged in farming and another 19.3% were indulged in petty trading while only 2.8% were involved in weaving as their means of living. This finding is consistent with GSS [25, 39] discovery that many people in both districts were illiterates and their main occupation is agriculture.

	Frequency	Percent (%)
Educational attainment		
No formal education	102	48.1
Basic	81	38.2
Secondary	20	9.4
Tertiary	9	4.2
Total	212	100
Occupation of respondent		
Farming	87	41
Petty trading	41	19.3
Housewife	34	16
Dress making	28	13.2
Weaving	16	7.5
Food vending	6	2.8
Total	**212**	**100**

Source: Field survey, 2019.

Table 1.
Educational achievement and occupational distribution of respondents.

5.2 Access to maternal healthcare

Access to maternal healthcare services was analysed first, on aggregate and later based on location. The results of the analysis show that 93.9% of the respondents had enrolled unto the national health insurance scheme whereas the rest had not registered to benefit from the exemption of pregnant women from paying the premium. Further analysis was conducted based on community of origin to determine whether differences exist with respect to enrolment unto the NHIS. The results indicate that 89.8% of the respondents had enrolled unto the NHIS in the Wa-East district, whereas 97.4% of them were registered with the scheme in the Wa-West district. This suggests that the Wa West district had more women registered under the NHIS than Wa East district. A chi-square test for independence (with Yates Continuity Correction) was carried out to determine whether there is an association between enrollment unto the NHIS and seeking maternal healthcare services. The test results revealed no significant association between registration for NHIS and seeking maternal health care [χ^2 (1, n = 212) = 0.00, p = 1.00, phi = −0.03]. This finding is in line with Twum et al.'s [7] discovery that in Ghana, pregnant women do not pay a premium for fresh registration or renewal of membership and processing fees.

We sought to find out whether respondent paid money to be registered under the NHIS in the sampled communities. The results showed that 75% of the respondents mentioned that they did not pay money to register under the scheme while the rest indicated that they paid money to register at the time they were pregnant. This means that the 25% who paid money to be registered under the scheme did not go to any health facility to confirm their pregnancy before they went for the NHIS registration. This is because a confirmation of the pregnancy is required by the NHIS to exempt a pregnant woman from premium payment. The results further indicate that in the Wa East District, 70.4% of the respondents noted that they did not pay money to be registered whereas the rest of them stated that they paid money to be registered. On the other hand, 78.9% of the respondents in the Wa West District reported that they did not pay money to register under the NHIS while the rest specified that they paid money to register under the NHIS. This hints that government expenditure on the exemption of pregnant women from paying the premium amount to the proposition of a key tenet of the access theory that concerns expending resources for individual/or collective benefit [4].

The distance of the nearest health facility from the sampled communities was considered. The results indicate that the minimum distance was 1 km whereas the maximum distance to the nearest health facility was 17 km with a mean of 6.5 (Median = 6.2; Quartile Deviation = 3; Skewness of 0.94) and an associated Standard Deviation of 5.22. The distance of the nearest health facility was also examined based on location and the results in the Wa East district indicate that the longest distance to the nearest health facility was 17 km while the shortest distance was 6.2 km and a median of 6.2 (Mean = 9.8; Std Deviation = 5.2 Skewness = 0.697) and with an associated quartile deviation of 5.4. However, in the Wa West District, the minimum distance to the nearest health facility was 1 km radius whereas the maximum distance was 12 km and a median of 1 (Mean = 3.7; Std Deviation = 3.2; Skewness = 0.41) with a related quartile deviation of 3. Comparing the medians, it is noticed that the median distance for Wa East is higher (6.2 km) than that of Wa West with a value of 1 km. This is inconsistent with Banik's [38] finding that the majority of pregnant women had their nearest health centre within a one-kilometre distance in Bangladesh. This difference is probably attributed to the variation in economic resources between Ghana and Bangladesh.

The amount of time spent travelling to a health facility to access healthcare has implication for the utilisation of services at the health facility. Therefore, the time spent to reach the nearest health facility was analysed first at the aggregate level and later based on location. The results indicate that the least time spent to reach the nearest health facility was 30 min or less whereas the maximum time spent was 3 h with a median of 45 min (Mean = 59.7; Std Deviation = 41.7; skewness = 1.54) and with an associated quantile deviation of 15. In the Wa East District, the maximum time spent to reach the nearest health facility was 3 h while the minimum time was 45 min and a median of 1 h (Mean = 86; Std Deviation = 42; Skewness = 1.18) and a corresponding quantile deviation of 45. On the contrary, the shortest time spent to reach the nearest health facility in the Wa West District was 30 min or less whereas the longest time was 2½ h and a median of 30 min (Mean = 43; Std Deviation = 25.9; Skewness = 2.92) and an associated quartile deviation of 15. Juxtaposing the medians, it is realised that the median time spent to reach the nearest health facility in the Wa East District is more than that of the Wa West District. This signals that women in the Wa East District spend more than travelling to the nearest health facility than their counterparts in the Wa West District. This finding contradicts Nussbaum [16] view that efforts should be geared towards removing obstacles that perpetuate differences, marginalisation or discrimination based on geographical locations to ensure equal access to resources.

Waiting time at the facility before respondents were attended to was also considered. On aggregate, the results indicated that the median time spent waiting was 1 h and the minimum time was 30 min or less, while the maximum time was 3 h (Mean = 62; Std Deviation = 35.31; Skewness = 1.15) with an associated quartile deviation of 30. The data was further disaggregated based on location. The results show that in the Wa East, the maximum time respondents waited to be attended to was 3 h whereas the minimum time was 30 min or less with a median of 1 h (Mean = 55.7; Std Deviation = 34.9; a skewness = 1.77) and with a related quartile deviation of 15 min. On the other hand, the longest time spent waiting to be attended to in the Wa West was 3 h while the least time was 30 min and a median of 1 h (Mean = 67; Skewness = 0.73; Std Deviation = 34.7) and a corresponding quartile deviation of 19. Matching the medians, it is noted that there is no difference in the amount of time spent waiting to be attended to at the health facility in the two districts. The time spent at the health facility could be a disincentive for women to seek maternal healthcare if they have other activities to undertake. This finding confirms Banik [38] calculation that majority of pregnant women had to wait for about an hour before being seen by the nurses or doctors in Northern Bangladesh.

5.3 Utilisation of maternal health services

The utilisation of antenatal care services helps reduce stillbirths and neonatal death as well as prevents and manage risk associated with pregnancy [5, 30]. In this respect, the utilisation of maternal healthcare services was analysed. On a whole, the results show that 98.6% of the respondents went for antennal care during the last pregnancy while the rest did not attend because they had not registered under NHIS. Out of the 98 respondents in the Wa East District, 99% stated that they attended ANC and 98.2% of the 114 respondents in the Wa West District mentioned they attended ANC. Further, we wanted to know whether respondents completed the compulsory ANC attendance. The results at the aggregate level indicated that 86.9% of the respondents completed the recommended ANC attendance, whereas the rest did not complete the required attendance. The data was further disaggregated based on district of origin to determine whether differences existed as regards ANC attendance in the two districts. The results showed that 79.6% of the respondents in the Wa East district completed the recommended four ANC attendances, while the rest did not. Conversely, 93% of the respondents indicated that they completed the four mandatory ANC attendances in the Wa West District while the remainder did not fulfil it. This compares with the findings made by Wang et al. [28] that the majority of pregnant women reported at least one antenatal care visit in Ghana.

WHO [30] notes that the early uptake of ANC services enables skilled health personnel to identify risk, prevent risk and manage pregnancy-related diseases as well as engage in health education and promotion among pregnant women. As such, it is important to know when the first ANC was initiated. The results (**Table 2**) indicate that 29.2% of the respondents initiated the first ANC attendance during the first month of the pregnancy while 24.5% of them initiated it during the second month of the pregnancy and another 18.9% started attending ANC during the third month of their last pregnancy. The results further showed that an accumulated 1.9% of the respondents initiated after the seventh month of their last pregnancy. This signals that the majority of the respondents sought antenatal care early. This implies that they are likely to avoid pregnancy related complications and have safe delivery. The results of the current study appear to disagree with the finding made by Kibusi et al. [8] that timing of the first ANC visit was also low and few women completed the recommended ANC visits.

The month of the pregnancy in which the first ANC was initiated was examined based on location. As shown in **Table 2**, 33.7% of the respondents in Wa East initiated ANC attendance during the first month of the pregnancy whereas 20.4% started attending ANC during the second month and another 13.3% of them initiated ANC visits during the third month of their last pregnancy and the rest started attending ANC from the fourth month forward. Similarly, in the Wa West District, majority of the respondents initiated ANC attendance during the first 4 months of their last pregnancy. The results noted that 28.1% of the respondents in the district mentioned that they initiated ANC during the second month of their last pregnancy whereas 25.4 started attending ANC during the first month and another 23.7% of them stated that they began attending ANC during the third month of their last pregnancy. The rest initiated their first ANC visit from the fourth month onwards. This hints that more women in Wa East District initiate early ANC attendance than their colleagues in the Wa West District.

	Aggregate		**Wa East**		**Wa West**	
Month	**Frequency**	**Percent**	**Frequency**	**Percent**	**Frequency**	**Percent**
First month	62	29.2	33	33.7	29	25.4
Second month	52	24.5	20	20.4	32	28.1
Third month	40	18.9	13	13.3	27	23.7
Fourth month	32	15.1	16	16.3	16	14
Fifth month	16	7.5	11	11.2	5	4.4
Sixth month	6	2.8	3	3.1	3	2.6
Seventh month	1	0.5	0	0	1	0.9
Eighth month	2	0.9	2	2	0	0
Ninth month	1	0.5	0	0	1	0.9
Total	**212**	**100.0**	**98**	**100**	**114**	**100**

Source: Field Survey, 2019.

Table 2.
Distribution of the first month ANC was initiated.

The NHIS policy exempts women from paying the minimum contribution to the scheme [23]. In this regard, it is vital to know whether pregnant women made payments before they sought antenatal care. The results indicated that 58.5% of the respondents mentioned that they did not pay for anything during antenatal care whereas a smaller proportion (41.5%) stated that they made payment during ANC attendance. The data was further disaggregated based on the district of origin. The results showed that 55.1% of the respondents in the Wa East district noted that they pay for services when they sought for antenatal care whereas the rest indicated that they did not pay for anything when they sought antenatal care services. As regards Wa West District, 70.2% of the respondents said that they did not pay any money during antenatal care while the rest mentioned they paid money during the time they attended antenatal care. This hints that more women in the Wa East District paid money for services during antenatal care than their counterparts in the Wa West District. The respondents indicated that they purchased items such as drugs, scan, and laboratory test. The results compare with the findings reported by Dalinjong et al. [10] that women still paid for drugs, supplies, and laboratory services including ultrasound scans in rural northern Ghana.

Access to maternal healthcare services entails the ability of women to obtain prenatal, antenatal, facility-based delivery and postnatal services [5, 37]. Therefore, it is important to know whether respondents delivered at a health facility. On aggregate, the results indicate that 66.5% of the respondents mentioned that they delivered at a health facility while the rest did not. With respect to the districts, the result show that 81.6% of the respondents in the Wa West District delivered at a health facility whereas the rest did not. On the other hand, 51% of the respondents in the Wa East District they delivered at a health facility against 49% of them who did not deliver at a health facility. This suggests that more women had facility-based delivery in the Wa West District than in the Wa East District. Kibusi et al. [8] findings that majority of the respondents delivered at health facilities under skilled attendants is consistent with the results of this study.

Those who did not deliver at a health facility mentioned reasons for their inability to deliver at the nearest health facility. The absence of health personnel at the facility at the time they were ready to deliver was cited as a prime factor. They indicate that when they were due to deliver, they made it to the health facility but upon arrival the health personnel were not at post to assist them deliver. Also, some respondents explicate that the time of delivery came at midnight and thus they could not wait and travel to the nearby health facility. Another set of respondents asserted that there was no means of transport to convey them to the nearest health facility. The quotation taken from field notes in the Wa West District illustrates the situation of some pregnant women:

> *"The unborn baby started disturbing me at about 2:30 pm and I reported it to my mother-in-law. Some few minutes later, she brought a tricycle to convey me to the nearest health facility (at Kataa) which is 6.2 km away from our community. Upon arrival at the health facility, we were informed that the health personnel were not at post to attend to us. We had to return to our community and I delivered just at the entrance to my room" [42-year old woman, July 7, 2019].*

The quotation shed light on the difficult situation some pregnant women had to go through to deliver their babies. This finding is in contravention of the key tenet of the access theory that maintains that individuals/or group such as pregnant women should be able to benefit from material objects, persons and institutions such as health facilities and personnel [18] without hindrance. This finding equally disagrees with the social justice theory that proclaims that all individuals including pregnant women have the right to societal benefits such as access to health facilities and in accordance with acceptable procedures, norms and rules that promote basic rights, liberties and entitlement of individuals and or groups as well as improves the situations of the disadvantaged within a society [13, 15].

Ghana introduced a free maternal healthcare programme (FMHCP) under the NHIS in 2008 to alleviate the cost burden associated with seeking maternal healthcare [7]. In this respect, it is crucial to know whether women incur cost in seeking delivery care at the health facilities. The result shows that 79.7% of the respondents indicated that they incur cost in seeking delivery care whereas the rest mentioned that they did not incur cost in seeking delivery care at health facilities. The data was further disaggregated based on district of origin. Out of the 98 respondents in the Wa East District, 68.4% mentioned they incur cost when seeking delivery care whereas the rest did not. Similarly, the results indicate that 89.5% of the 114 respondents stated that they incurred cost when they sought delivery care while the rest did not in the Wa West District. According to the respondents, the cost element includes soap, sanitary pad, hand gloves, detergents, blade, bucket, and rubber sheet. This signals that more women in the Wa West district incurred cost during delivery compared to their counterparts in the Wa East District. This finding contradicts the assertion that health insurance protects the poor in particular against the risk of incurring medical and related financial costs at the point of service utilisation [9].

The cost involved in seeking delivery care was, therefore, examined. The cost here does not include service cost but rather the cost of detergents (Dettol antiseptic, soap and parozone bleach) and other materials such as rubber, blade, hand gloves etc. The detergents are usually collected by the health facilities from the pregnant women and used to clean and disinfect the labour ward after delivery. The least cost involved in seek delivery care was GH¢10.00 whereas the highest was GH¢400 with a median of GH¢40 (Mean = 57.64; Std Deviation = 69.23; Skewness = 3.4) and a related quartile deviation of 17.5. The data was further disaggregated based on location and the result indicated that in the Wa East District, the maximum cost was GH¢400.00 while the minimum was GH¢10.00 with a median of 35 (Mean = 59.55; Std Deviation = 82; Skewness = 3.5) and with an associated quartile deviation of 12.5. On the other hand, the lowest cost involved in seeking delivery care in the Wa West District was GH¢10 whereas the highest cost was GH¢345.00 and a median of GH¢45 (Mean = 56.60; Std Deviation = 61; Skewness = 3.06) and a corresponding quartile deviation of 18. Balancing the medians, it is realised that the median cost in Wa West is higher than the median cost in Wa East. Also, a Mann-Whitney U Test was conducted to test for differences in the cost of delivery care in the two districts. The test revealed no significant difference in the cost of seeking delivery care for Wa East ($Md = 35, n = 45$) and that of Wa West ($Md = 45, n = 82$), $z = -0.715, p = 0.475$. This finding agrees with Dalinjong et al. [10] assertion that pregnant women still purchase certain items for childbirth under the free maternal health policy in rural Northern Ghana. However, some of the respondents admitted that the cost of these items required for delivery sometimes deters them from going to the health facilities for delivery due to the high poverty levels in the study areas. This partly explains why some women still deliver at home.

Charlotte et al. [33] intimated that PNC ensures continuity of care for mother and baby as well as helps to support healthy behaviours. Thus, PNC contributes to the beneficial health outcome for the baby and the mother [5]. In this regard, it is important to know whether women continued seeking PNC. The results of the study noted that 91.5% of the respondents mentioned that they attended PNC while the rest stated that they did not attend PNC. In addition, the data was disaggregated based on location and the results indicate that majority of the respondents (81.6%) in the Wa East District attended PNC but the rest mentioned that they did not. In the Wa West District, however, all respondents stated that they attended PNC. The results of this study contradict the discovery made by Twum et al. [7] that women did not go for postnatal care. The probable reason for the difference in these findings is that our study area is rural where the nurses visit the communities for PNC whereas Twum et al. [7] conducted their study in an urban setting.

Health insurance coverage appears to provide a window of opportunity to reduce or eliminate Out-of-pocket expenditures at the point of service utilisation [17]. In this regard, it is prudent to determine whether women incurred cost when seeking PNC. The results denoted that 75% of the respondents stated that they did not incurred cost while the rest mentioned they expended money when they sought for PNC. Furthermore, the data was segregated based on location to determine whether differences exist between the districts as regards cost incurred during PNC. The results showed that in the Wa East District, 68.4% of the respondents stated that they did not incur cost when they sought for PNC while the rest mentioned that they expended money. As regards the Wa West District, majority (80.7%) of the respondents indicated they did not make payment during PNC whereas the rest signalled they incurred expenditure. Those who admitted they made payments alluded to contribution to construct a delivery room and paying for the security of the health facility.

The person who makes the decision to seek maternal healthcare tends to influence attendance. As such, it is crucial to know whether the wife alone, the husband only or a joint decision influenced the utilisation of maternal healthcare services. The results (**Table 3**) indicate that majority of the respondents (54.2%) mentioned that it was the wife who initiated the decision to seek maternal healthcare services while 24.5% of them indicated that the decision was jointly made by the husband and wife. The data was also disaggregated based on district of origin to determine whether differences exist between the two districts. The results show that 35.7% of the respondents in the Wa East District indicated that it was the wife who took the initiative while 34.7% mentioned that the decision was jointly made. With respect to the Wa West District, 70.2% of them indicated that the decision was taken by the wife and another 15.8% stated that the man and wife jointly took the decision to seek maternal healthcare services. This finding does not fall in line with that of Banik [38] who reported that decisions about seeking maternal healthcare services made by both husband and wife were higher compared to those made by husband or wife alone. The contradiction in these findings could be due to cultural differences between Ghana and Bangladesh.

	Aggregate		Wa East		Wa West	
Spouse	**Frequency**	**Percent**	**Frequency**	**Percent**	**Frequency**	**Percent**
Wife	115	54.2	35	35.7	80	70.2
Joint	52	24.5	34	34.7	18	15.8
Husband	45	21.2	29	29.6	18	14
Total	**212**	**100**	**98**	**100**	**114**	**100**
Source: Field Survey, 2019.						

Table 3.
Distribution of decision about seeking maternal healthcare services.

6. Conclusions and policy implications

Health insurance coverage appears to contribute to improved access and utilisation of maternal healthcare services. In this respect, majority of the respondents had enrolled unto the NHIS in both districts even though some pregnant women paid for the registration and renewal of their cards which was inappropriate since it was supposed to be free for them. Equally, women largely sought for antenatal and post-natal care during pregnancy and after delivery respectively. Furthermore, some pregnant women incurred cost at the point of registration or renewal of their NHIS cards. Still, some pregnant women deliver at home due to lack of transport, unavailability of health personnel, and the timing of delivery. In addition, a significant proportion of the pregnant women who sought delivery care spend money to purchase certain items at health facilities or from the market before they are admitted to deliver. Moreover, the decision to utilise maternal healthcare services was made mostly by the women themselves.

Together, a number of steps can be taken to ensure the full realisation of providing free maternal healthcare to all women. First, it will be prudent for the government to station at least one trained health personal particularly midwives in all communities to provide delivery services to pregnant women. Second, the government, through the District Health Directorate should provide the basic items that are needed to provide safe and smooth delivery at the health facilities. Third, the communities should be encouraged to provide a communal means of transport to convey pregnant women who are due for delivery to nearby health facilities. Fourth, management of the NHIS in collaboration with the health personnel should embark on continuous sensitization of women on the need to always visit a health facility to confirm their pregnancy before they register or renew their NHIS cards so as to benefit from the free maternal healthcare policy of government. Above all, the District Health Directorates should monitor the movement of health personnel to ensure that at least one personnel (especially the Midwives) is always at post to provide maternal health services for women.

Acknowledgements

We indebted to our research assistants, Mr. Josephat Derbile and Mr. Galaa Mwinbuobu Vitus who are teaching assistants in the Department of Governance and Development Management of the University for Development studies for their hard work and commitment during the data collection stage of the study. Indeed, you demonstrated commitment in spite of the short time we had to collect the data. We are grateful to you. We are also thankful to Dr. Moses Naiim Fuseini and Afia Dankwah Dentaa of the School for Development Studies, University of Cape Coast for proof reading the manuscript and offering invaluable suggestions to help improve the manuscript.

Conflict of interest

We wish to declare that none of the authors have any conflict of interest in connection with this study.

Author details

Ibrahim Abu Abdulai and Abdul-Moomin Adams*
Department of Governance and Development Management, University for Development Studies, Tamale, Ghana

Address all correspondence to: adamsmoomin@gmail.com; amadams@uds.edu.gh

IntechOpen

© 2019 The Author(s). Licensee IntechOpen. This chapter is distributed under the terms of the Creative Commons Attribution License (http://creativecommons.org/licenses/by/3.0), which permits unrestricted use, distribution, and reproduction in any medium, provided the original work is properly cited.

References

[1] Devaux M. Income-related inequalities and inequities in health care services utilisation in 18 selected OECD countries. The European Journal of Health Economics. 2013;**16**:21-33

[2] Terraneo M. Inequalities in health care utilization by people aged 50+: Evidence from 12 European countries. Social Science and Medicine. 2014;**126**:154-163

[3] Moscelli G, Siciliani L, Gutacker N, Cookson R. Socioeconomic inequality of access to healthcare: Does choice explain the gradient? Journal of Health Economics. 2018;**57**:290-314

[4] Ribot JC. Theorizing access: Forest profits along Senegal's charcoal commodity chain. Development and Change. 1998;**29**(2):307-341

[5] Rutaremwa G, Wandera SO, Jhamba T, Akiror E, Kiconco A. Determinants of maternal health services utilization in Uganda. BMC Health Services Research. 2015;**15**(1):271

[6] Krůtilová V. Unmet need for health care—a serious issue for European elderly? Procedia - Social and Behavioral Sciences. 2016;**220**:217-225

[7] Twum P, Qi J, Aurelie KK. Effectiveness of a free maternal healthcare programme under the National Health Insurance Scheme on skilled care: Evidence from a cross-sectional study in two districts in Ghana. BMJ Open. 2018;**8**:e022614. DOI: 10.1136/bmjopen-2018-022614

[8] Kibusi SM, Sunguya BF, Kimunai E, Hines CS. Health insurance is important in improving maternal health service utilization in Tanzania—Analysis of the 2011/2012 Tanzania HIV/AIDS and malaria indicator survey. BMC Health Services Research. 2018;**18**(1):112

[9] Ho A. Health Insurance. Encyclopedia of Global Bioethics. 2015:1-9

[10] Dalinjong PA, Wang AY, Homer CS. The implementation of the free maternal health policy in rural Northern Ghana: Synthesised results and lessons learnt. BMC Research Notes. 2018;**11**(1):341

[11] Abduali IA, Adams A, Abdulai M. Seeking healthcare under the National Health Insurance Scheme's capitation payment method in Wa Municipality, Ghana: Subscribers' perspectives. African Journal of Science, Technology, Innovation and Development. 2018;**11**(1):45-54

[12] Loewen G, Pollard W. The social justice perspective. Journal of Postsecondary Education and Disability. 2010;**23**(1):5-18

[13] Jost J, Kay AC. Social justice: History, theory, and research. In: Fiske ST, Gilbert D, Lindzey G, editors. Handbook of Social Psychology. 5th ed. Vol. 2. Hoboken, NJ: Wiley; 2010. pp. 1122-1165

[14] Robeyns I, Brighouse H. Introduction: Social primary goods and capabilities as metrics of justice. In: Robeyns I, Brighouse H, editors. Measuring Justice: Primary Goods and Capabilities. Cambridge, MA: Cambridge University Press; 2010. pp. 1-13

[15] Bankston CL. Social justice: Cultural origins of a perspective and a theory. The Independent Review. 2010;**15**(2):165-178

[16] Nussbaum MC. Creating Capabilities: The Human Development Approach. Cambridge, MA: The Belknap Press, University of Harvard; 2011

[17] Lagarde M, Palmer N. The Impact of user fees on access to health services in low-and middle-income countries. Cochrane Database of Systematic Reviews. 2014;(4)

[18] Ribot JC, Peluso NL. A theory of access. Rural Sociology. 2003;**68**(2):153-181

[19] World Health Statistics. Monitoring Health for the SDGs, Sustainable Development Goals. Geneva: World Health Organization; 2018. Licence: CC BY-NC-SA 3.0 IGO. Available from: https://apps.who.int/iris/bitstream/handle/10665/272596/9789241565585-eng.pdf [Accessed: 03 June 2019]

[20] World Health Organization. Pregnancy, childbirth, postpartum and new-born care: A guide for essential practice. Geneva: World Health Organization; 2015

[21] Government of Ghana. National Health Insurance Act, 2012 (Act 852). Accra: Government of Ghana; 2012

[22] Andoh-Adjei FX, Boudewijns B, Nsiah-Boateng E, Asante FA, van der Velden K, Spaan E. Effects of capitation payment on utilization and claims expenditure under National Health Insurance Scheme: A cross-sectional study of three regions in Ghana. Health Economics Review. 2018;**8**(1):17

[23] Ghana Health Service. Family health division 2015 annual report. Accra: Ghana Health Service; 2016

[24] Ghana Statistical Service (GSS), Ghana Health Service (GHS), ICF. Ghana Maternal Health Survey 2017: Key Indicators Report. Accra, Ghana: GSS, GHS, and ICF; 2018

[25] Ghana Statistical Service. 2010 Population and Housing Census: District Analytical Report, Wa West. Accra: Ghana Statistical Service; 2014

[26] Ghana Health Service. Upper regional health service 2016 annual report. Accra: Ghana Health Service; 2017

[27] Wa East District Assembly. The Composite Budget of the Wa East District Assembly for the 2016 Fiscal Year. Accra: Ministry of Finance; 2016. Available from: https://www.mofep.gov.gh/sites/default/files/composite-budget/2016/UW/Wa-East.pdf [Accessed: 03 June 2019]

[28] Wang W, Temsah G, Mallick L. The impact of health insurance on maternal health care utilization: Evidence from Ghana, Indonesia and Rwanda. Health Policy and Planning. 2016;**32**(3):366-375. DOI: 10.1093/heapol/czw135

[29] World Health Organization. Fact Sheets on Sustainable Development Goals: Health Targets. Antimicrobial Resistance. 2017. Available from: http://www.euro.who.int/__data/assets/pdf_file/0006/354921/3.1-SDG-Fact-sheet-Maternal-Health.pdf?ua=1 [Accessed: 08 June 2019]

[30] World Health Organization. Neonatal and Perinatal Mortality: Country, Regional and Global Estimates. Geneva: World Health Organization; 2016

[31] Lincetto O, Mothebesoane-Anoh S, Gomez P, Munjanja S. Antenatal care. In: Opportunities for Africa's newborns: Practical data, policy and programmatic support for newborn care in Africa. The Partnership for Maternal, Newborn and Child Health. 2006. pp. 51-62

[32] Demott K, Bick D, Norman R, Ritchie G, Turnbull N, Adams C, et al. Clinical guidelines and evidence review for post natal care: Routine post natal care of recently delivered women and their babies. London: National Collaborating Centre for Primary

Care and Royal College of General Practitioners; 2006

[33] Charlotte W, Pat D, Lalla T, Pyande M. Postnatal care. In: Opportunities for Africa's newborns: Practical data, policy and programmatic support for newborn care in Africa. The Partnership for Maternal, Newborn and Child Health; 2006. pp. 79-90

[34] Timilsina S, Dhakal R. Knowledge on postnatal care among postnatal mothers. Saudi Journal of Medical and Pharmaceutical Sciences. 2015;**1**:87-92

[35] Aday LA, Anderson RM. Equity of access to medical care: A conceptual and empirical review. Medical Care. 1981;**19**:4-27

[36] Gulliford M, Morgan M, Hughes D, Beech R, Figeroa-Munoz J, Gibson B, et al. Access to health care. Report of a scoping exercise for the National Co-ordinating Centre for NHS Service Delivery and Organisation R&D (NCCSDO). London: NCCSDO; 2001

[37] Ganle JK, Fitzpatrick R, Otupiri E, Parker M. Addressing health system barriers to access to and use of skilled delivery services: Perspectives from Ghana. The International Journal of Health Planning and Management. 2016;**31**(4):235-253

[38] Banik BK. Barriers to access in maternal healthcare services in the Northern Bangladesh. South East Asia Journal of Public Health. 2016;**6**(2):23-36

[39] Ghana Statistical Service. 2010 Population and Housing Census: District Analytical Report, Wa East. Accra: Ghana Statistical Service; 2014

[40] Yamane T. Statistics: An introductory analysis. NY, USA: Harper & Row; 1967

[41] World Health Organization. Women and Health: Today's Evidence, Tomorrow's Agenda. Geneva: World Health Organization; 2009

Section 2

Significance of Hygiene: Current and Future Perspective

Chapter 3

Comparative Assessment of Hygiene Behaviour Change and Cost-Effectiveness of Community Health Clubs in Rwanda and Zimbabwe

Juliet Anne Virginia Waterkeyn, Regis Matimati, Andrew Muringaniza, Agrippa Chigono, Amans Ntakarutimana, Joseph Katabarwa, Zachary Bigirimana, Julia Pantoglou, Anthony Waterkeyn and Sandy Cairncross

Abstract

Two similar Community Health Club (CHC) interventions to achieve hygiene behaviour change and improved family health in Africa took place—one in Zimbabwe implemented by an NGO and the other in Rwanda as part of a Randomized Control Trial. Both interventions achieved high levels of community response, although the Zimbabwe project was more cost-effective, achieving blanket coverage of all households in the area with over 90% compliance in 12 recommended practices at a cost of US$4.5 per beneficiary in 8 months. In Rwanda, the spread of the intervention reached only 58% of the households in the first year costing US$13.13 per beneficiary. By the end of three years, the spread had increased to 80% with over 80% of the 4056CHC Members adopting 10 new practices without any extra cost to the project. Although the Zimbabwe program showed better Value for Money, being more efficient, long term sustainability to prevent slippage of hygiene behaviour change depends on a strong monitoring system. Scaling up hygiene behaviour change is best achieved systematically by building the capacity of the Environmental Health Department to take responsibility for the supervision of CHCs in every village. Investing in an integrated national program, which can enable Government to coordinate NGO efforts, is a more cost-effective use of scarce resources in the long term.

Keywords: community health clubs, cost-effectiveness, hygiene behavior change, Zimbabwe, Rwanda

1. Introduction

With a strong international drive to achieve the Sustainable Development Goals (SDGs) and end absolute poverty by 2030 [1] there is a renewed interest to broaden community development initiatives from the 'silo vision' which characterized much community development from 2000 to 2015, when the Millennium Development Goals (MDGs) [2] encouraged a more narrow focus, to a more integrated approach with the current SDGs. As no single SDG goal on its own will be sufficient to completely eliminate poverty, implementing organizations are looking for ways to combine programs across sectors: for example, the Goal 6 (Safe Water and Sanitation) if combined with Goal 2 (Food Security and Good Nutrition), is likely to be more successful in improving Goal 3 (Improved Family Health). If, in the same program, Goal 5 (Women's Empowerment) results in Goal 8 (increased Employment), then a substantial reduction of the primary Goal 1, (the elimination of *Absolute* Poverty) would be expected. Integrated programs are not only more aligned with this holistic people-centered approach but will also be more likely to be cost-effective.

The Community Health Club (CHC) model of community development is an integrated and holistic strategy to start up CHCs—voluntary Community-Based organizations (CBOs) in rural or peri-urban area—which include all residents in active membership of a group. Membership of a CHC is freely available to all ages, education levels and social status. The club meets weekly for at least 6 months to find ways to improve family health by preventing common diseases through safe hygiene, with the purpose of increasing social capital, through shared understanding and coordinated action with the objective to improve living standards with existing resources.

The CHC is the vehicle for community development which, if extended into a full A.H.E.A.D Model (Applied Health Education and Development), can easily coordinate many activities into a single program in a process of development in four main stages, preferably over a 4-year period:

- Stage 1: Health Promotion (HP): Health education and participatory activities to improve hygiene (Goal 3)

- Stage 2: Water, Sanitation & Hygiene (WASH): construction of facilities through self-supply (Goal 6)

- Stage 3: Food, Agriculture and Nutrition (FAN) Clubs: nutrition gardens and ensuring a balanced diet (Goal 2)

- Stage 4: Gender Equity & Women's Empowerment (GEWE): management of income generating projects (Goal 5 and 6)

2. The development of the Community Health Club Model

2.1 Community health clubs in Zimbabwe

In Zimbabwe, the Community Health Club (CHC) Model of development has succeeded in mobilizing communities in over 2340 CHCs in an integrated way (mainly Stages 1 and 2) over the past 25 years, through Africa AHEAD, the pioneer of this approach, thereby benefitting over 1.7 million people, across over half the districts in the country [3]. Although the full four-stage AHEAD Model has been used less often due to sector-specific donor funding in past years, the full AHEAD model was successfully conducted in 285 CHCs in Makoni District between 1999 and 2003 [4] and was found to be a cost-effective method of integrated development at <US$5 per beneficiary per year for Stage 1. Since 2003, over 30 NGOs have

been trained by Africa AHEAD and CHCs are now routinely used throughout Zimbabwe by most NGOs. CHCs have enabled many communities to be better organized to mitigate against cholera [5] as well minimize common diseases such the diarrhea, pneumonia and malaria, skin and eye diseases as well as neglected tropical diseases such as intestinal helminths (worms) and schistosomiasis (bilharzia) which were virtually eliminated in reported clinical cases in an area in Makoni District where CHCs had been active for 4 years [6]. An assessment of hygiene behavior change in CHC programs in Chipinge, Chimanimani and Buhera Districts also showed a strong pattern of hygiene improvement based on monitoring records of the program, where 12,311 CHC members enrolled in 127 FAN Clubs [7]. This resulted in improved livelihoods and social capital through communal nutrition gardens with a community member reporting: '*There was a new spirit of cooperation, empathy and love within the participating communities as a result of the FAN intervention as the training provided a mechanism for visiting each other and showing empathy for each other in times of need.*' Although there is much anecdotal evidence through qualitative research [8–10] in Zimbabwe, there is an absence of any comparative research on CHC impact and 'Value for Money' between different countries in the published literature.

2.2 Replication of the CHC model to other countries

Africa AHEAD was instrumental in starting CHCs in around 20 countries through the training of other NGOs. Project monitoring records of these initiatives have shown positive hygiene behavior changes in a diverse range of cultures. In East Africa, an outstanding response was recorded in Uganda in 2004, where 116 CHCs were started in 15 camps for internally displaced people enabling the construction of 8504 latrines, as well as 6060 bath shelters and 1552 hand washing facilities within 4 months [11]. In peri-urban areas in both Namibia [12] and South Africa [13], CHCs have been successfully used to enable community maintenance for ablution facilities in informal settlements. In one South African slum, open defecation was reduced by 76%, and dumping of solid waste reduced by 50%. In the rural areas of Kwa Zulu Natal, communities improved their hygiene, sanitation and water supply through CHCs [14].

In West Africa, the Community Health Club Model was introduced into Sierra Leone in 2002 for post conflict rehabilitation, which then morphed into the 'For Di Pikin Dem Wel Bodi' program which is successfully improving child and maternal survival rates in Koinadugu District [15]. CHCs were also used to mobilize Muslim communities in a trial in Guinea Bissau to reduce infant and maternal mortality by increased treatment seeking behavior [16].

The CHC concept was transplanted from Africa to the urban slums in the Caribbean, firstly being replicated into the Dominican Republic [17], and then, more successfully, across the island to Haiti by voluntary community leaders who report that CHCs '*foster positive social relations that can positively improve health-related behaviors* [18].' In Guatemala they are being used to build trust to enable a strong community response for a water supply project [19]. In 2009, Vietnam, the Ministry of Health started CHCs in three provinces which they considered a '*low cost, high impact*' method demonstrating a significant reduction in diarrhea cases as measured by reported clinical cases at a cost of under one dollar per CHC beneficiary using government environmental health workers [20].

However, none of these programs have been revisited to assess their progress nor have different programmes been compared in published literature and much useful learning is being lost for lack of such research.

2.3 Scaling up the Community Health Club Model in Rwanda

Rwanda is the only country in Africa to have embedded the CHC model into a national program known as the Community Based Environmental Health Promotion Programme (CBEHPP) [21]. In 2010 the Economic Development and Poverty Reduction Strategy II laid out the target of *'CHCs with enhanced health promotion and behaviour change capacity'* to reach 70% of all villages in Rwanda by 2018 [22]. By 2015, CBEHPP had succeeded in establishing CHCs in virtually all the 15,000 villages throughout this small, but highly organized country of 12 million people. CBEHPP contributed to Rwanda becoming one of only five countries in Africa to meet sanitation targets of the MDGs and to halve the number without sanitation in the country. The *Imihigo* assessment is a regular evaluation by government in Rwanda whereby each Mayor is held accountable for various achievements (including a CHC in every village). The *Imihigo* assessment in 2015 recognized that CBEHPP had successfully galvanized communities in Rusizi District to achieve hygiene and sanitation change [23].

Based on the Rwandan success story using CBEHPP, the African Union (AU), with backing from the African Development Bank (AfDB) and the African Ministers' Council for Water (AMCOW) recommended in 2016 that the CHC Model should be used in the 10 most fragile states in Africa to achieve the SDGs. The AU's Kigali Action plan states:

'... Rwanda has gained substantial experience with social approaches such as the Community Based Environmental Health Promotion Programme (CBEHPP) and Community Health Clubs (CHCs) the implementation of which has enabled the country to significantly reduce the debilitating national hygiene and sanitation-related disease burden and, in so doing, attain key outcomes in efforts to achieve the MDG targets not only for water supply and sanitation, but also poverty reduction outcomes.' [24].

CBEHPP in Rwanda, having reached most villages across the country, has now been extended into a well-resourced USAID-funded Integrated Nutrition–WASH program which aims to reduce the prevalence of stunting in eight districts using existing CHCs to roll out a Food Security and Nutrition program in line with the 'full' four-stage AHEAD Model, thus providing a valuable example of CHCs being taken to scale.

3. Cost effectiveness

The rationale for providing water and sanitation initiatives has been based on the need to control diarrheal diseases, which still claim the life of one in every nine children before their fifth birthday [25]. Whilst many diseases can be fairly easily controlled by a single action (e.g. the use of insecticide treated bed-nets to prevent malaria), the control of diarrhea is more challenging because there are at least five main transmission routes through which feces reach the mouth. These are known as the '5 "F's"– Flies, Fluids, Fingers, Food, and Fields [26] - all of which have to be safely controlled if the prevalence of diarrhea is to decease. It has long been understood that if only one "F" component is addressed alone, without the other 4 "F's" then diarrhea is unlikely to be successfully reduced. Research has shown that safe drinking water is estimated to reduce diarrhea by only 15%, safe sanitation by 35%, hygiene promotion by 33% [27] and regular handwashing with soap by 47% [28]. The training in the CHC tackles all 5 "Fs" over a 6 month period and therefore theoretically (if over 80% of CHC members respond and improve their hygiene) diarrhea should be decreased.

However, diarrhea accounts for only 11% of death globally among children under five in developing countries: pneumonia accounts for 18%; complications during pregnancy for 14%; death in childbirth 9% and malaria for 7% of child deaths [25]. The most effective intervention to prevent infant deaths would be to improve nutrition because malnutrition (miasma) accounts for 33% of all the deaths mentioned above i.e. Children who have pneumonia, diarrhea, and malaria have less chance of survival if they are malnourished and stunted. Many of these child deaths could be prevented with little cost, if mothers were properly trained in CHCs, enabling them to improve their understanding of disease prevention, to protect their children by safer hygiene in the home and ensure early treatment to reduce child mortality.

However, there is a caveat – as public health relies on reaching the critical mass in a population, we maintain that at least 80% of the CHC members should conform to the recommended practices if any impact is to be found on prevention of diarrhea. This critical assumption is highlighted in the recent debate [29, 30] as to whether CHCs in Rusizi District in Rwanda, achieved sufficient quality and quantity of training to bring about the prevention of diarrhea let alone control stunting.

Although much research has been done in WASH literature on a *single* aspect of 'effectiveness' (i.e. water *or* sanitation *or* hygiene) there are few peer reviewed papers that address *all three* of these essential aspects of WASH. This may be because few programs are sufficiently integrated to *provide* all three inputs. A review of a Cost-Effectiveness Analysis [31] found only six studies, of which, only three, met the minimum level of methodological soundness. Two of these referred to our own work in Zimbabwe [4, 32] and the other to a study in Bangladesh [33]. In this review, 'Effectiveness' was defined as '*the adoption of specific recommended hygiene practices by those exposed to a health promotion programme*', whilst '*Cost*' was calculated roughly by taking the monetary expense of only the *field* inputs divided by the number of people benefitting, giving a '*cost per person per year*'. In this paper we use the same definition of 'cost-effectiveness' as it is measured in monetary terms (US$) – i.e. the production of '*a unit of effect through an intervention*'. The term 'Value for Money' is similar but emphasizes the *quality* of services.

This paper looks at the cost-effectiveness of two interventions which use the CHC Model: an intervention in Rusizi district in Rwanda implemented between 2014 and 2017 which was part of the National CBEHP Programme, and a project in Mberengwa District in Zimbabwe implemented in partnership with an NGO between 2012 and 2014. We access the different inputs and analyze the cost-effectiveness of the two different strategies against intermediate outcomes of hygiene behavior change.

The field cost includes all training expenses of personnel but does not include costs of directs inputs in the form of subsidy for cement for sanitation nor water hardware, i.e. filters or handpumps. Neither were the indirect costs for the NGO management nor research costs included in this calculation of cost-effectiveness. Indirect beneficiaries, (i.e. those outside the program that might benefit incidentally by diffusion of innovation or emulation) were not counted, as we only monitor the households who are registered CHC members and their immediate family living within the household (defined as 'those eating from the same pot').

4. Description of the interventions

4.1 Mberengwa District, Zimbabwe

The CHC approach in Zimbabwe has been adopted into both the National Water Policy [34] and the National Sanitation and Hygiene Policy [35], although the Government of Zimbabwe has not yet been able to launch a national CHC program to coordinate the sector as has been so effectively done in Rwanda. In Zimbabwe, NGOs are largely coordinated through UNICEF which heads the WASH Cluster. Zimbabwe AHEAD (ZA) partnered with Action Contre la Faim (ACF) to implement the Public Health Promotion and Community Livelihoods Improvement Program in Gutu and Mberengwa Districts [9]. Midlands Province is one of the most arid areas of Zimbabwe with a low rainfall of 150–250 mm. Literacy is over 80% for both men and women. ZA was responsible for the 'software' (meaning mobilization and training of people) in Stage 1 (Health Promotion), whilst ACF managed the implementation of the 'hardware' component (i.e. infrastructure) for the Stage 2 (Water and Sanitation) and Stage 3 (Food, Agriculture & Nutrition) (FAN) in the two subsequent years.

The main task for ZA was to mobilize the community and to start up and train CHCs, in order to promote full community participation and inculcate increased responsibility to ensure strong community ownership for the water provision programme. Most people in the area are subsistence farmers, but as many men are away from home all year working in South Africa, their wives remain to run their farms. The year 2012 was not an enabling period in which to run a program in a remote rural area, as the economy had collapsed with hyperinflation, political tensions were high, and Zimbabwe had dropped to the 14th lowest in Human Development Index in the world [36] with a critical scarcity of fuel, banknotes and electricity.

Stage 1 of the program ran for 24 months, from February 2012 to January 2014. This was a well-staffed programme with 6 field officers stationed across 8 wards, supervised by a programme manager based in the District Office (**Table 1**). The aim was to achieve blanket coverage of households in these wards, so that all available households were within in a CHC.

Unlike other CHC programmes where CHCs have around 100 members, ACF was adamant that to ensure better quality of training, the size of the CHC membership should be restricted to between 40 and 50 members in each CHC. Therefore, to enable the whole village to join, a second CHC would be formed if there was enough demand from the community. In fact, such was the popularity of the CHCs that the target of 8208 possible members was exceeded with a total of 9615 members registered resulting in universal coverage within 2 years (**Table 1**). To achieve more gender balance, it was strongly advocated by the project officers in mobilizing the community, that the CHC was not only a woman's concern, but that husbands as well as wives should be members. As a result, there were 1196 male CHC members (18% of the total membership), resulting in 1407 households where both husband and wife attended the CHC together. Blanket coverage was achieved with the total number of members being 17% more than number of households. As for compliance with training, with sufficient time and personnel, all of the CHCs managed to complete the required number of 20 training sessions, with 4864 sessions being held in total. Mberengwa had an exceptional completion rate, with 77% of CHC members graduating with full attendance, which is higher than many other CHCs project in Zimbabwe.

Ministry of Health had three Environmental Health Technicians (EHTs) stationed in the project area who were meant to be involved in the programme but had no transport: they relied on the NGO which effectively managed the program, with all field officers having their own motorbike. To understand the scale of the project, mobilization details can be compared between Mberengwa in Zimbabwe and Rusizi in Rwanda (**Table 1**).

4.2 Rwanda: Rusizi District

In 2012, a cluster Randomized Controlled Trial (cRCT) was proposed to establish the cost-effective of the CHC model within CBEHPP. Rusizi District was

	Rusizi, Rwanda		Mberengwa, Zimbabwe	
Mobilization targets	**Actual achieved**	**Expected target**	**Actual achieved**	**Expected target**
# Community Health Clubs (CHC)	50	50	243	237
Average # of members/CHC	81	70	40	34.6
# households in all villages	6942	n/a	8208	n/a
Mean of family in a household	4.7	n/a	4.4	n/a
# CHC members in all CHCs	4056	5000	9615	8208
Ratio female: male members in CHC	58:42	60:40	80:20	60:40
% of CHC coverage in a village	63%	80%	117%	100%
Number beneficiaries (family)	19,063	23,500	42,595	36,115
# NGO field officers in field	1	1	6	6
# Motor bikes for NGO field officer	0	2	6	6
# Environmental Health Officers	10	50%	3	6
# Motorbikes for MoH	5	50%	0	0%
# Weeks of training	16	24	24	24
# Health sessions held in all CHC	718	1200	4860	4860
Mean # health sessions / CHC	14.5	24	20	24
Mean attendance of members /CHC / session	41	50%	26	34
Literacy level women (men)	73%	n/a	80 (85%)	80%
# (%) of CHC members graduating	1703	42.4%	6335 (77%)	8208
Cost of Project (field costs only) US$	250,325	n/a	193,529	n/a
Cost in US$ per beneficiary	13.13	5	4.5	5
Cost in US$ per family	61.71	25	22	25

Table 1.
Comparative summary of community mobilization of 50 classic villages in Rusizi District, Rwanda in 2014 with 243 classic CHCs in Mberengwa District, Zimbabwe in 2012.

selected for the intervention as it was one of the least developed areas of Rwanda with one of the highest levels of diarrhea and stunting in the country. There were 79,880 households in 596 villages with a total population of 375,436. Most of the population are subsistence farmers or fisherman with some trading across the nearby border to Burundi and the Democratic Republic of Congo [37]. The total population for the 50 Classic villages was 32,313 people within 6866 households, with an average of 646 people and 137 households per village, and an average of 4.7 people per household. Literacy is 73% for men and women over the age of 15 [38]. Rusizi has a tropical climate and rainforest with heavy annual rainfall of over 1400 mm per annum, with most falling between February and May.

The start-up of the CHC intervention was delayed by 6 months whilst the baseline and randomization of villages was being completed. By November 50 CHCs were formed (**Table 1**), one in each intervention village. The engagement of village leaders in the start-up was neglected due to difficulty with transport as the short rains had already just begun, making many villages inaccessible in tropical mountainous terrain. Nevertheless, the intervention was expected to continue despite the season, and facilitators were selected and trained in February 2014. Training took place from March to June during the long rains, and the period was curtailed to 5 months when the intervention had to wind up activities according to the research protocol. For a full one year after the training ended (July 2014 to June 2015), the cRCT permitted no follow up by project implementation staff: there was no opportunity for revision of sessions, no model home competitions and very few graduations held as promised to reward those who had completed the training. After this year, without any external support to the community, the post intervention survey for the cRCT was undertaken. It was estimated that the intervention had only a 54% fidelity to protocol [30].

Of the possible 6942 households in the 50 villages, 4056 were enrolled in CHCs (50.7%) and of these 3144 CHC members (62.8%) attended weekly sessions with 42.4% competing all 20 sessions. Due to shortage of training period, and lack of monitoring and supervision by Ministry of Health, only 10 CHC came near to meeting mobilization targets: 76% had over 100 CHC members, only 50% reached over 80% coverage of households in a CHC in 1 year. Only 6% of CHC met the required target of providing 20 sessions of training within the intervention period—the mean being 14 meetings. The average attendance of all registered members at CHC sessions was 41 members per meeting. Although the 10 Environmental Health Officers had been expected to implement the intervention, they were grounded with no transport for the duration of the project. Africa AHEAD had only one monitoring officer but she did not have a dedicated vehicle, having to hire a motorbike taxi to monitor the whole district of 960 sq.km of challenging terrain during the heavy rains [30].

4.3 Methodology of training in a community health Club

The CHC methodology of training in both Zimbabwe and Rwanda is considered to be the 'Classic' CHC training (**Table 2**): although the CBEHPP Manual [40] was adapted to the Rwandan context, it was based on the original manual produced by the architects of the approach in Zimbabwe in 2009 [39]. In both countries CHC facilitators are given visual aids known as a 'Tool Kit" of illustrated A5 cards, which help to stimulate discussion in a variety of activities. CHC facilitators are usually nominated by the village leader from each village. They are voluntary and do not receive any financial incentives for the time they give the community although they receive basic equipment (a T-shirt, hat, boots, rucksack, raincoat and possibly a bicycle). CHC Facilitators are then trained by Ministry of Health extension staff or by the implementing NGO in a five-day training workshop, during which they acquire participatory facilitation skills as well as learning the transmission routes and basic information about prevention of common diseases addressed in the various sessions When the facilitator returns to the village she registers as many members as possible to form up a CHC with a member from every household in the village and issues each member with a membership card (See CHC. **Figure 1**).

A health club can be compared to a religious group or a Scout meeting which assembles regular members together every week for a couple of hours. With a program to address local health and hygiene challenges, the regular opportunity to gather provides much team-building with songs and slogans that help to reinforce the knowledge which is gained through the 'dialogue sessions'. Much use is made of key messages in visual aids, as well as being acted out in drama and role play. 'Participatory activities' such as the '*Three pile sorting*', or '*Blocking the Route*' activity are used to engage members. These games were originally developed to engage community in the 'Participatory Hygiene and Sanitation Transformation' (PHAST) training methodology for the maintenance of water and sanitation facilities [26].

The CHC aims to produce a cohesive community where there is genuine 'common-unity' of understanding, belief and practice. The group itself makes the rules which influence individual behavior and practices similar to the iterative process of peer learning pioneered in the education sector [41]. Each topic focuses on a *single*

	Key components of a classic CHC intervention	Zimbabwe classic	Rwanda classic
1	District Ministry of Health (MoH) is fully involved/ supportive/funded directly	Yes	Partially
2	Politically enabling environment through a national policy	Yes	Yes
3	A CHC Manual, customized to national conditions	Yes	Yes
4	A tool kit of culturally appropriate visual aids	Yes	Yes
5	All sessions are participatory/dialog not didactic	Yes	Yes
6	24 × 2 h participatory sessions are provided	Yes	Partially
7	One topic per session with a recommended preventive practice	Yes	Partially
8	CHC Facilitator is local volunteer/Community Health Worker	Yes	Yes
9	All CHC facilitators have a thorough 5 day training	Yes	Yes
10	Environmental Health Officers monitor CHC and assist facilitator	Yes	10 EHOs but no transport
11	Enough dedicated NGO Project Officers (PO) supports MoH monitoring	Yes. 10x POs	No. Only 1 PO
12	24 session last for 6 consecutive months in dry season	Yes	4–5 months in wet season
13	All members have a membership card signed on attendance	Yes	Yes
14	A certificate is awarded at a graduation ceremony for full attendance	Yes	Not all CHCs had graduation
15	Monitor with household inventory at base and end line	Yes	Yes
16	Model Home Competitions held at the end of training	Yes	No, none held
17	There is no material subsidy for water/sanitation	Yes	Yes
18	CHCs aim to have 50–100 members who are registered	Yes	Yes
19	CHCs aim to have >50% members complete all 24 sessions	Yes	Yes
20	Household Coverage of CHCs in a village should be over 80%	Yes	Only 10% of CHC reached 80%

Table 2.
Specifications for a Classic CHC Intervention, showing fidelity to protocol in Zimbabwe and Rwanda interventions.

aspect of hygiene, with a *single* activity recommended as homework, which does not incur much cost for the household (e.g. covering stored drinking water, constructing a pot rack). Incremental change is seen gradually over time, but it is our belief that at least 24 sessions over 6 months are needed to be sure that knowledge and practice are sufficiently reinforced (**Figure 1**).

CHC members receive no material incentives or food for attending health sessions, and the lack of "hand-outs" is made clear at the start of the program, ensuring that there are no false expectations of material gain. Despite this lack of material incentive, CHCs invariably attract a consistently high attendance rate at health sessions over an extended period, and there has seldom been any difficulty attracting a large crowd of 50–100 people in the many projects discussed above.

A membership card is given to each member when they join the club (**Figure 1**). This card gives confidence to members that the facilitators will provide the specified number of sessions, so providing a psychological guarantee that the training will, in fact, be completed. Members appear to value their membership cards highly

	Topic of the Session	Homework for the session
1.	What is a Community Health Club	Bring Friends and family next time
2.	Common Preventable Diseases	Be able to identify preventable disease
3.	Superbugs (antimicrobial resistance)	Build a handwashing facility
4.	Handwashing & Personal Hygiene	Build a family bath shelter
5.	Skin Diseases (Scabies & ring worm)	Ensure all kids treated for skin disease
6.	Diarrhoea/cholera, dysentery)	Clean up the yard regularly
7.	Infant Care & Immunisation	Ensure all kids are immunised
8.	Intestinal Parasites (worms)	Treat all kids for skin disease
9.	Food & Kitchen Hygiene	Build a pot rack for drying plates
10.	Nutrition & Balanced Diet	Start having a balanced diet
11.	Food Security & Food processing	Build a food drying rack
12.	Protected Water Sources	Ensure protected water source
13.	Storage/handling of drinking water	Ensure containers clean & covered
14.	Safe & Hygienic Sanitation	Ensure zero open defecation
15.	Solid Waste Management	Separate, Recycle and Reuse waste
16.	Safe Environment Management	Woodlot/fruit tree/organic fertilizer
17.	Safe Animal Management	Management of parasites & waste
18.	Criteria for a Model Home	All of the above, in each home
19.	Good parenting /child development	play with kids each day
20.	Youth issues (alcohol/drug abuse)	Talk to teenagers about their issues
21.	Combatting Malaria	All use insecticide treated nets
22.	Pneumonia	Correct use of antibiotics
22.	Bilharzia (schistosomiasis)	Don't go in infected water
23.	Combatting HIV/AIDs & Tuberculosis	Abstain, one partner or use condom
24.	Fertility and Reproductive Health	Know contraceptive methods

Figure 1.
Inside of a typical membership card showing topics and homework for each session.

keeping them carefully wrapped in plastic at home like their cards from a clinic. They enjoy the challenge of completing their cards, by attending all sessions [8]. They are then rewarded with a certificate, and this aspect of the CHC model may be the key to high attendance rates.

Seeking to understand the popularity of the CHCs, we found from interviewing CHC members in Zimbabwe that the principle attraction of CHCs, is their perceived need for knowledge, especially related to the health and wellbeing of their family. This love of learning appears to be one of the principle drivers of the CHC Model [8].

4.4 Context of the two interventions

The key components for a CHC intervention were very similar in both Rusizi and Mberengwa, aiming to meet all the specifications for the 'Classic' CHC Training (**Table 2**). In both interventions the key messages in 24 topics on the Membership Card were similar and local villagers were used as community-based facilitators to run the weekly health sessions, whilst Environmental Health Staff were expected to help *monitor* the intervention whereas in Rusizi they were meant to *implement* the program. An important difference between Zimbabwe and Rwanda, is that whereas the Mberengwa project was *community-led* and could expand to respond to the demands of the CHC members, being unconstrained by programme length or design, the Rwandan programme in the Rusizi trial was tightly controlled by the *research* protocol and had no flexibility to adjust timing or scope as the end line survey had to be completed before registered toddlers grew out of the cohort.

Hygiene and sanitation standards between the two countries vary considerably. In Zimbabwe the Government recommended standard for sanitation is a Blair Ventilated Improved Pit (BVIP) latrine which usually has brick lined pit with cement slab, whilst the superstructure is likely to be permanent constructed in bricks, often plastered with cement with a tin roof and vent pipe with a fly gauze at the top to trap flies, thereby preventing breeding, as well as reducing smell.

For many years the building of BVIP latrines for the community was extensively subsidized by NGOs in WASH programs in Zimbabwe, but with the political turmoil and resultant socio-economic collapse of the country in 2000 when most donors withdrew, there has been little sanitation subsidy. As a result, the high coverage of improved sanitation which climbed rapidly during the 1990's and reached over 63% by 2000, had, a decade later, plummeted to around 25% in most areas, with a return to much open defecation [42]. Without such support, householders tended to build temporary latrines until they could afford the better standard of a BVIP. Instead of a brick wall and tin roof householders would sometimes use traditional mud and pole for walls with a thatch roof to save costs, but invest in lining the pit, having a cement slab and most importantly a vent pipe as is shown in **Figure 2** above. Research shows that it is the cost of a BVIP that prevents quicker uptake, but that with time CHC members do aim for this high government standard [43]. If they cannot afford to construct a proper latrine, CHC members are encouraged to practice 'cat sanitation' (i.e. the burial of their feces in a hole). This simple method is in fact more hygienic than an uncovered pit latrine which can add to the spread of diarrhea by becoming a breeding site for flies. A hand washing station known as a 'Tippy tap' is common practice in Zimbabwe, made from a jerrycan strung from local branches with a foot operated method for tipping out water.

In Rwanda, over 90% of households have their own latrine and there is little defecation in the surrounding bush [30]. The superstructure is usually made of mud/pole walls and thatch roof. The norm is an unlined pit latrine, with poorly fitting logs with gaps between them, straddling the pit and the smell is always unpleasant and there are frequently feces on the floor (See **Figure 2**). As the pit is not properly sealed flies breed in great numbers and the pits are often thick with maggots making this method highly unsanitary. This could be called 'fixed point open defecation' as it is no more sanitary than open defecation on the ground. The level of handwashing with soap is extremely low in Rwanda, and there are seldom handwashing facilities outside such latrines although most households have soap and wash hands in a common bowl before eating.

Zimbabwean households usually have a dedicated kitchen with an open fireplace in the centre of the round thatched cooking hut. Seating for men is a molded bench around the walls, whilst women and children sit on the ground by the fire, and chickens enter freely. The hut is usually very smoky causing a high rate of acute respiratory infections (See **Figure 2**). Traditionally, cooking huts were highly decorated with built-in clay shelving in the walls and this practice has been reinvigorated by the CHCs with all members upgrading their kitchens in ever increasing levels of excellence.

Water is stored in well covered containers and food is kept in containers to protect from flies and rodents. Many now use fuel-efficient stoves built in clay, and have seats for women on a par with men, thus showing increased gender equity. All food and utensils are stored in this kitchen hut which is kept locked (**Figure 3**).

Cooking in Rwanda, as in many East African countries, is done outside on an open fire (**Figure 3**). There is no culture of a dedicated kitchen hut as in Zimbabwe, and therefore the storage of utensils is haphazard, with no special place to store cooking pots, plates or food. Sometimes this is kept in the main house in boxes or baskets but almost always open to vermin. There is usually a shelter outside where goats are tied and this often doubles to provide shelter for cooking in the rains. Water is collected in a jerry can and stored unsystematically often without a cover. Filtration of water and fuel-efficient stoves are being promoted by government but uptake is still relatively low.

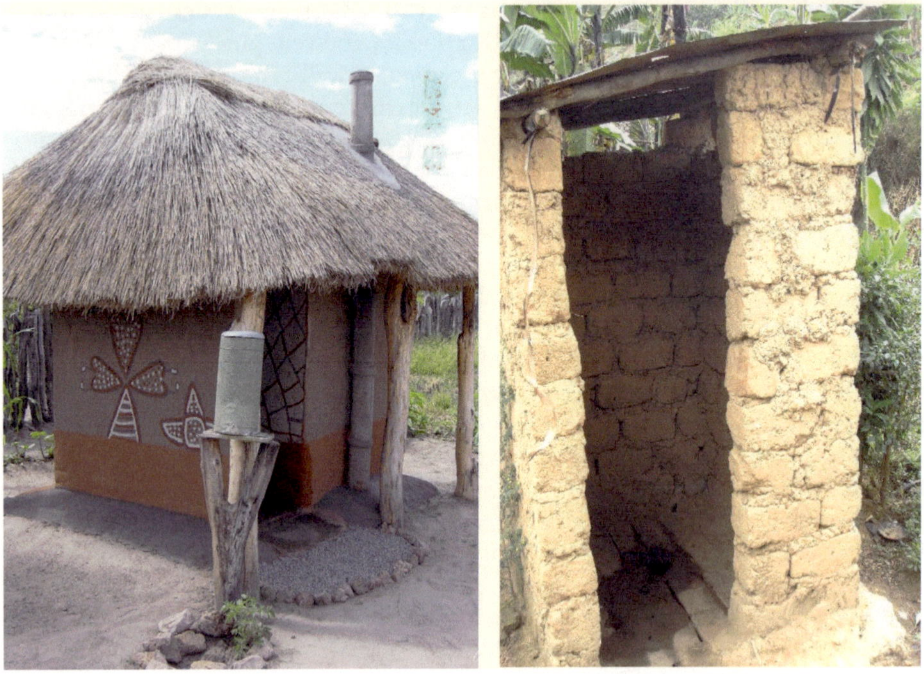

Figure 2.
Left: Subsidized ventilated improved pit latrine (VIP) in a CHC home in Zimbabwe with lined pit, concrete slab and vent pipe - a fly trap which eliminates smell and a hand washing facility. Right: An unsubsidized traditional pit latrine in Rwanda, unlined and open pit, log floor giving open access for flies. Photographs courtesy of J. Waterkeyn.

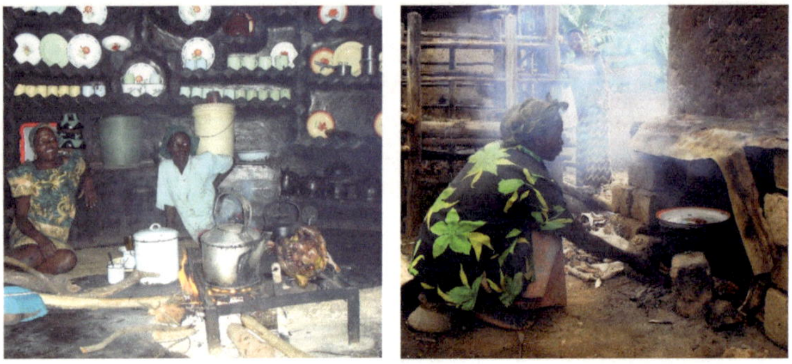

Figure 3.
Left: A model CHC kitchen hut in Zimbabwe showing shelving made of clay, individual family utensils and covered drinking water with ladle. Right: In Rwanda, a traditional cooking shelter outside, with no CHC improvements. Photographs courtesy of J. Waterkeyn.

5. Methods

5.1 Data collection

5.1.1 Popularity

Popularity of the CHC can be measured by the ability of the facilitators to attract many members and retain their attendance for the duration of the intervention. The Membership Cards of all members were collected at the end of the training and this was triangulated with project records to ascertain overall number of members in the intervention, percentage of households within a CHC in each village and number of members completing the training i.e. graduating. This enabled us to have exact numbers of *active* members to calculate cost per beneficiary.

5.1.2 Effectiveness

Effectiveness was demonstrated by the *community response to the training* as measured by the percentage of members adopting each of the recommended practices. The observation check list, known as the *'Household Inventory',* was used to conduct spot surveys which uses proxy indicators of hygiene behavior change which can be empirically observed first-hand by the enumerator. We did not use self-reported data as we are skeptical of the value of this method given the well-known effect of observer bias. For example: although we can observe the presence of handwashing facility (HWF) and whether soap was present, the calculation of regular usage over time is not observable. To overcome this monitoring challenge, all members are required to place a pot plant beneath their HWF. If the pot plant has been regularly receiving water from the HWF, and is alive, we know the HWF is likely to be in use. Similarly, we do not place much credibility on reported behaviour, as householders when asked this question, are likely to answer that they are in compliance with handwashing methods and use soap. To avoid such interviewer bias, we simply ask a child to demonstrate how they wash their hands and we note whether soap is used. Observations in Rwanda were conducted by Environmental Health Officers (EHOs) and trained enumerators drawn from teachers and students for a random selection of CHC member households. In Zimbabwe CHC facilitators, CHC chairpersons and Environmental Health Technicians (EHTs) collected data.

5.2 Data analysis

5.2.1 Quantitative analysis of cost-effectiveness

Project Records and accounts were used to ascertain field costs. An Analysis of Cost-Effectiveness was done by dividing the field costs by number of direct beneficiaries within a one-year time frame and was calculated, giving a 'cost per direct beneficiary per year' for improved hygiene [31]. Direct beneficiaries are taken to be all those within the household of a CHC Member, estimated at 4.7 people per household in Rwanda, and 4 people per household in Zimbabwe based on local census.

5.2.2 Analysis of community response: hygiene behavior change

In Rwanda a custom-made digital application for mobile phones was designed for CBEHPP which enabled data to be entered directly online thus eliminating most human error, through instant processing online using Open Development Kit (ODK) a free application for data analysis. This data was downloaded into in excel and then analyzed in SPSS.

In Zimbabwe the data was collected by Project Officers and CHC facilitators and entered into excel computer program manually and analyzed in excel to generate a bar chart of before and after (at least 6 months after training) for each program.

5.2.3 Qualitative analysis of value for money

In Rusizi, the results were provided to all stakeholders involved in the training with Ministry of Health and 25 EHOs through Focus Groups Discussions at District Level. The EHOs were asked to identify and discuss reasons for the variation between CHCs and to provide contextual rational for some of the anomalies, or where targets were under or over-reached. These insider observations from the grass roots provides the explanation for various challenges and shortcomings, as well as reasons for success of the CHC Model allowing some recommendations to achieve better Value for Money in future CHC programs based on the CHC Theory of Change [30].

In Mberengwa, an in-depth observation was taken on a small sub-set of six CHCs using an interpretivist approach. This was triangulated with participant observation, key informant interviews and focus group discussions involving Environmental Health staff, local leaders, CHC members and others. Field work was done over 2 weeks in Ward 19, which had 39 CHCs in the 43 villages and a population of 9245, in 1481 households. In addition, two villages without CHCs were sampled to serve as control groups to enable comparison [10].

5.3 Limitations and possible sources of bias

We use project monitoring data which, we accept could be open to interviewer bias as the field officers who managed the programme also assisted the facilitators in the collection of the village data. However, an effort has been made to minimize this bias, by using an external researcher in each country to clean data, excluding all incomplete data and verifying all records and findings in Rwanda [32, 45] and Zimbabwe [44] through spot observations. It is also not ideal that all that co-authors of this paper have been associated either with the design of the CHC approach and the implementation of the intervention in both Zimbabwe and Rwanda and may not be strictly impartial. However, in the interests of our genuine concern to improve learning in the sector, we have attempted to provide only such programming evidence which has been verified by external observers conducting research for their own theses which have subsequently been properly peer reviewed.

6. Results

6.1 Mobilization of community

6.1.1 Mberengwa District, Zimbabwe

The completion rate of the CHC training was exceptionally high in Mberengwa with full attendance of all 20 sessions by 6335 (77%) of CHC members. With sufficient time to repeat many of the session for a second time, all members had the opportunity to complete the training if they had missed the original session due to other commitments. The CHC training was well-timed by the NGO to coincide with the dry season (March – December 2012) to coincide with the 8 months of the year when there is little demand from farming to distract members from the training. All CHCs did more than 20 sessions properly, providing only one topic only per session of at least 2 hours of participatory activities. All the mobilization targets were not only achieved but surpassed during the first year, with follow-up by Project Officers, who arranged model home competitions. All CHC held their Graduation ceremonies properly with CHC members receiving certificates with due recognition. Those who did not finish in Year 1 had a second chance to complete their training and graduate in Year 2, while the water and sanitation component of the project was being done. However, as the number of members was limited to 50 per CHC, we could not judge the popularity of a CHC by the number of members in the normal size of CHCs as is routinely expected in Zimbabwe, where CHC can reach over 100 people. Instead we ascertain the level of popularity by the fact that there was universal coverage with over 1407 households (17%) having two members in the CHC. Therefore, the CHC model in Mberengwa was clearly very popular.

6.1.2 Rusizi District, Rwanda

The completion rate of the training in Rwanda was not as high as had been hoped with only 41% of CHC members attending all 20 sessions in 5 months. However, this appeared to be, not because they did not *want* to attend sessions, but because they did not want to get wet in the torrential rain! In addition, the training was held during the season that farmers were at their busiest in the fields, planting and weeding crops. Not as many members completed as was expected because the training was shortened by a full month and they had no opportunity for repeating any sessions. Crucially there was no time for Graduation Ceremonies and no "Model Home competitions" were held as had been planned. However, monitoring records show that in the post research intervention, all CHCs continued to meet and over 6 sessions were done per CHC after the official end of the cRCT [30]. This demonstrates the demand for CHC activities. As attendance continued without external support, we would take this as an indication of a high level of sustainability. In Rusizi District, despite the constraints encountered by the community, the large size of the CHC in terms of memberships with an average of 80 members per CHC which exceeded the expected target of 70 members per CHC demonstrates popularity of the CHC. At the end of the cRCT intervention (i.e. after the first year), the spread of the intervention had only reached 58%. However, by the end of 3 years, the spread of CHC households had increased to 80% with CHC members ranging from 40 to 100% in 50 villages.

Our monitoring data shows that the uptake of the CHC model in Rusizi, although it was slow initially, did eventually meet all targets. Therefore, we would consider the CHC project to be a popular intervention in Rusizi District, and that what appears to have been community resistance was mainly due to external constraints imposed by the research and implementing team. Once Ministry of Health had clearly endorsed the intervention, the village leaders whole heartedly led the CHC with much interesting anecdotal evidence of community-led initiatives.

6.2 Hygiene behaviour change

6.2.1 Mberengwa District, Zimbabwe

The household observation included 7477 households in the end line survey (**Figure 2**) in Mberengwa District, with a clear pattern of community effort being evident in all indicators ($p > 0.001$).

Of the 21 indicators, 12 were found in over 90% of CHC households, and three indicators were found in over 80% of households after 8 months. To measure the effect of the CHC it is important to note which indicators have made the most change. The most impressive change from baseline to the post intervention 8 months later, was in the use of hand washing facilities in the home which increased by 85.4% (from 6.4 to 91.8%), the use of ladles to draw water from a bucket increased by 65% (18–83%), bathing rooms increased by 51% (16–67%), the use of pot racks to dry plates increased by 51% (46–97%), the use of refuse pits to ensure fly control increased by 39% (58–97%), decorated kitchens increased by 30% (66–95%), Blair Ventilated Improved Latrine (BVIP) for a household increased by 27% (from

14–41% households), the use of protected water sources for drinking water increased by 23% (61–84%), ventilation of housing increased by 21% (65–86%). Use of mosquito nets whilst still low (8.9–19.8%) increased by 11% and fuel-efficient stoves increased by 14% (4.2–18.2%) (**Figure 4**) [46]. The effect of the improved hygiene could be quantified by the condition of the children. Over 90% of CHC households could demonstrate children with no skin diseases, no worms, and a complete immunization card for all children. Mothers in over 90% of CHC homes could demonstration how to treat dehydration with a Sugar salt rehydration solution.

It is noteworthy that changes which required purchasing were on the lower end of the scale with BVIP latrine construction, buying mosquito nets and fuel efficient stoves being the least amount of change. As this was during a time when Zimbabwe was completely dysfunctional economically and while there was over 75% unemployment in the country, with over 3 million Zimbabweans living abroad as economic migrants, it is not surprising there was little affordability. Indeed given this context it is impressive that 2108 high quality BVIP latrines which cost at least US$100 at the time (when cement was in short supply nationally) were built by self-supply by households in some of the most challenging areas in the country.

After only 8 months, the post intervention survey showed that compliance level was over 80% of the registered CHC members in 15 indicators (**Figure 4**), of which 12 were over 90%, which leaves little doubt as to the effectiveness of the CHC training to stimulate exceptional levels of community response in Mberengwa District.

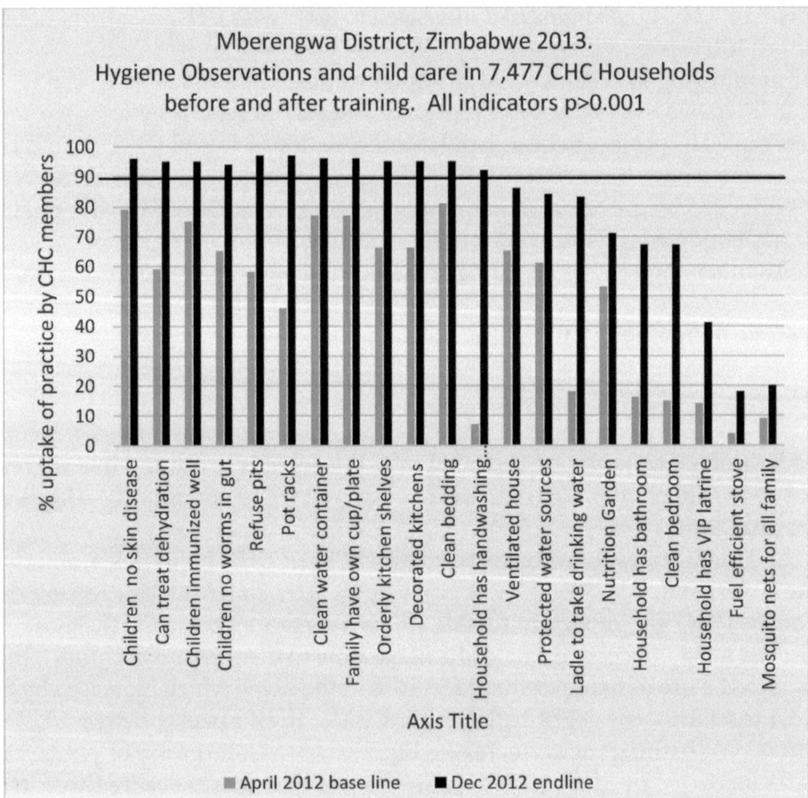

Figure 4.
Percentage hygiene behaviour change of 7477 CHC members in Mberengwa District, Zimbabwe. 2012 [46].

6.2.2 Qualitative study

In one ward of Mberengwa a qualitative study was conducted in three villages [10] which established that CHC members were considerably more knowledgeable than non CHC members. Understanding the cause of diseases was claimed by CHC members to be the reason for their increased use of safe borehole water and the construction of latrines raising coverage in a village from 36.6–53%, and hand washing facilities by 22.1% (from 5 to 27.1%).

The study states in the conclusion,

> *'As community members reflected on the impact of CHCs on their lives, the increases in their health knowledge was evident and participatory practices were prevalent across the CHCs. CHCs are currently bringing about a multitude of positive change, as the activities initiated by their members are practiced at the community level. Not only have health indicators changed, but more importantly, village member's perceptions of their capacity have increased; they feel more able to control disease and improve their lives. More importantly, they are taking action to prevent disease and sharing what they have learned with other communities' [10]*

6.2.3 Rusizi District, Rwanda

Safe hygiene correlated positively in all but three of the 24 indicators with the number of sessions attended by members (p-value <0.001) (**Figure 5**).

To demonstrate an impact on sanitation in Rwanda was complicated by the fact that four of the indicators did not change significantly simply because, even *before* the start of the intervention, compliance was already exceptionally high - meaning little

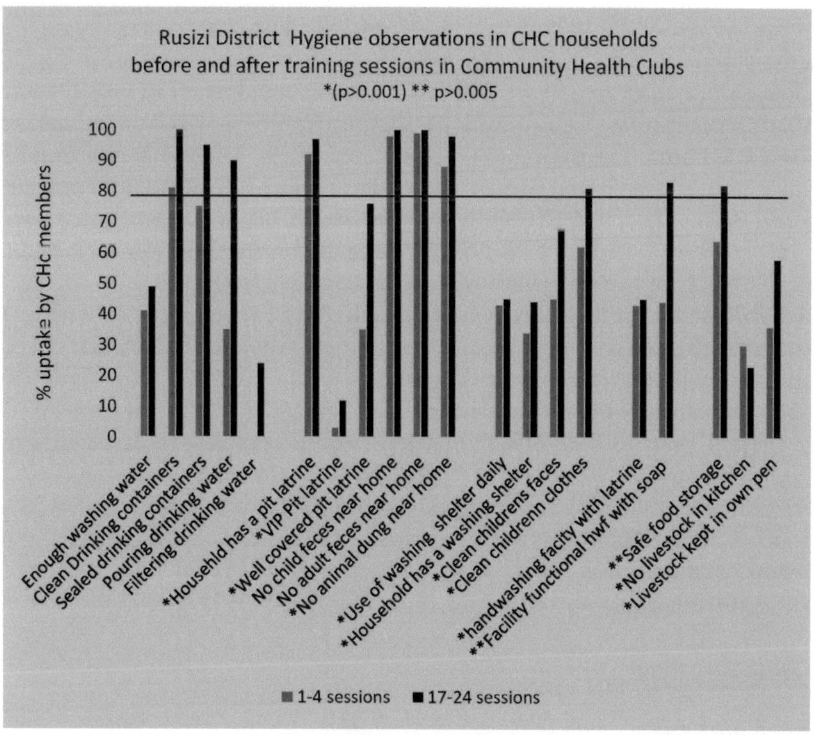

Figure 5.
Percentage hygiene behaviour change of all CHC in Rusizi District, Rwanda. 2017 [45].

improvement could be expected as a result of the CHC training: 91% of households already had their own latrine, 98.5% households showed no child feces, 99.6% showed no adult feces and 90% showed no animal feces in the yard. With this exceptionally high level of latrine ownership, sanitation indicators were altered after the baseline, to an observation of the *hygienic standard* of the open pit latrines, with the recommendation that there should now be a well-fitting foot-operated cover for the squat hole to prevent fly access and breeding. Monitoring data showed a 40% increase in '*having and using a well-fitted cover for the squat hole of latrines*' which increased from 35.5 to 76.5% [46]. The indicator "cover for the squat hole" is the most important indicator of the research, because unlike all other indicators, it was completely unique to the intervention and therefore unlikely to be confounded by previous initiatives [46] (**Figure 4**). This indicator showed that a 41% uptake of covered squat holes may be taken as a proxy indicator of the effect of the CHC on hygiene practice.

Thirteen of the most important indicators showed a significant increase of $p > 0.001$ (Pearson Chi-Square Asymptomatic Significance) and these are strong indicators of the high level of compliance shown by CHC members in relation to the training: a 5-fold uptake increase from those attending only 1–4 sessions as compared to those who have completed 17–20 sessions [45].

The quality of drinking water has been improved by a combination of improved practices for serving drinking water: 18% more households were making sure that jerry cans used to store drinking water were clean inside (81.9–100%) and that they were closed with lids (from 76.1–95%). A massive rise of 55% in the non-risk practice of the family taking drinking water by *pouring* from a jerry can rather than *dipping* into an open container (34.8–90%) would also decrease risk of contamination of drinking water in the home. The practice of using a (plastic) water filter increased by 24.2% from zero to 24.2% of families who had taken advantage of a district wide distribution of water filters to increase safe water consumption in Rusizi District [45] (**Figure 5**).

Personal hygiene improved slightly with the construction of more bath shelters in yard that increased by 10% (from 34.1 to 44.1%). The construction of a Tippy Tap in the yard increased by 35% (48.3–83.3%) as functional hand washing facility (with soap) were observed, of which 45.3% were situated near latrines. Overall child cleanliness increased enormously with the awareness of the danger of flies spreading Trachoma. The data show 23.1% increase (50–73.21%) in children having clean faces as indicated by no flies on their faces although this gain was not sustained and reverted back to 52.6%. In an increased effort to prevent skin diseases, CHC mothers were washing children's clothes more often. Children with clean clothes on the day of the observation increased by 18% from 63.3 to 81.3% but then dropped to 76.3%, Although this indicator could have been associated with muddier clothes during the wet season [45] it is clear that mothers need continual encouragement to keep their children cleaner (**Figure 5**).

Most importantly for the transmission of germs by the fecal oral route, the 'safe storage of food' improved by 24% from 63.6 to 81.8%, but also recessed later to 71.8% [45] (**Figure 5**).

As regards the prevention of zoonotic diseases, 22% of households (36–58%) had constructed livestock pens away from the kitchen area, and less animal dung was seen in 7% more yards (88.3–90.9%) which were free from animal dung, decreasing further ingestions of germs spread by flies [45] (**Figure 5**).

6.2.4 Qualitative study

A small qualitative study [47] was also conducted in two CHC Villages in Rusizi District and compared with two non CHC villages to ascertain the perception of the community towards the CHC project.

> *'They testify to have seen the difference between villages with and without CHC and that 90% of sanitation and hygiene improvement can be achieved through CHC implementation. Community members appreciate the strategies of the CHC approach as it raised spontaneously project initiatives and tangible achievements including, but not limited to, making roads, proper nutrition through balanced diet, mutual assistance, saving and loans and tontine strategies, Kitchen garden, water treatment, as well as being a role model in the community. The village members of Kakinyaga and Kareba villages not exposed to CHC activities wish to have CHCs and think their sanitation and hygiene practices would improve through CHCs. Community members of the exposed villages confirmed CHC implementation facilitated mutual assistance so that even vulnerable households can have sanitation and hygiene facilities. "We have been engaged more with CHC and we believe everything is possible" said the head of village of Nyambeho and the president of the CHC committee in Kanyetabi separately. During the focus group discussions, the following was the statement in Rusizi: "we have been always sick but CHC has been a solution to prevent hygiene related disease." [47]*

As the CHC model in CBEHPP was being implemented by around 15 NGOs in Rwanda, there was data from monitoring programs in other Districts such as Bugasera [48] where experience by WaterAid confirmed extensive community response [49] reinforcing much of the positive community feed-back received in Rusizi District. When the disappointing result of the cRCT in Rusizi was presented at the 3rd national CBEHPP Conference in 2017, experienced practitioners of CBEHPP were skeptical of the results as the findings did not tally with other experience of CHC outputs in Rwanda. At the same time the cautious academic conclusion of the cRCT was questioning 'the value of implementing this intervention at scale with the goal of improving health outcomes', the MoH was convinced that the CHC model worked and government was expanding the programmes into the Integrated Nutrition and WASH Program which was to use CHCs in 8 new districts to address stunting with support from UNICEF and USAID [50].

6.3 Comparative cost-effective analysis of Rusizi and Mberengwa districts

6.3.1 Rusizi District, Rwanda

In Rusizi District, the cost of implementing the cRCT intervention in 50 villages over 12 months amounted to US$208,204. These costs were for the setting up of the intervention, and interface with the community, with the main activity being the training and monitoring of 50 CHCs. It was a very low budget operation with only a small support staff in the country (one field officer, one monitoring officer in Kigali, a part time programme manager and an accountant) with minimal support of external consultants. With a total of 4056 CHC members in the Classic Villages we calculate 19,096 beneficiaries i.e. family members in the household who have benefited directly from improved living conditions over 50 different indicators. The program is calculated to have cost US$13.13 per beneficiary or US$ 61.71 for an average family of 4.7 people. This figure does not include research costs of the cRCT Evaluation costs.

6.3.2 Mberengwa District, Zimbabwe

In Mberengwa District, the cost of the whole programme for 1 year was one fifth less expensive than the Rwandan intervention, at US$193,529 for a programme of 1 year, which reached five-fold more CHC villages, and with 42,959 beneficiaries had twice as many beneficiaries as Rwanda. The costs included the operational support for 6 field officers and a programme manager, with part time administrative costs for the organization headquarters in Harare, and a shared office in the field. The program is estimated at only US$4.5 per beneficiary, or US$22 per household.

7. Discussion

7.1 Spread of the intervention

The two case studies show that the most successful villages are those where high level of diffusion of innovation has taken place with at least 80% of the households being included within a CHC. Mberengwa District achieved blanket coverage and were able to show over 90% uptake across most indicators. In Rusizi, it was found that villages which had less than 100 households were able to achieve 80% CHC training across all households in the village but only after 3 years. This is a realistic target if sufficient personnel and transport are available to run the program to its best level. The *size of CHCs* seems less relevant than the importance of reaching *all households* in a village, within one or two CHCs. In small villages of under 100 households this can realistically be achieved in the first year, but larger villages need another year to achieve blanket coverage. Perhaps a standard target would be 70 households per year per CHC facilitator. This shows that *village size* should be considered when selecting intervention area so as not to over work each facilitator. A critical mass is likely to be more successful to prevent the spread of diseases such as cholera and diarrhea and malaria, and so this becomes the ultimate test of effectiveness.

7.2 Quality of the intervention

The cost-effectiveness of a program depends not only on the Value for Money it can achieve (i.e. how *many* benefits it can deliver, and the *quality* of those benefits), but also on the way the program makes the most of scarce resources and takes advantage of *economies of scale*. The more CHCs that each officer can supervise the less the cost for personnel. We have seen that the size of a CHC can vary from 30 to 100 people. Although Mberengwa demonstrates that a greater number of smaller CHCs (with around 40–50 members) may be more manageable, this may not be the most cost-effective method, as the more people per CHC facilitator, the less the program will cost per beneficiary. Typically, an EHO should be able to monitor one or two CHCs per day, traveling constantly between villages. Therefore, the most cost-effective design is to have at least 100 CHCs in a program monitored by 10–20 EHOs, depending on the transport. Critically, each EHO should have a motorbike with a dedicated fuel allowance, supplied directly to the district.

7.3 Dedication of Environmental Health staff

While EHOs in both countries showed complete personal commitment, they were almost always frustrated by the lack of transport in the Ministry of Health, preventing such staff from reaching out and supporting Community Health Club facilitators in distant villages. Those CHCs which were situated near where Environmental Health Officers resided did much better than those in remote villages which were left to their own devices. Although the CHC enables even poorly educated facilitators to run the CHC, they do need strong support from the Ministry of Health with regular back-up of Environmental staff monitoring.

7.4 The importance of transport

The investment in transport is one of the key inputs required for a health promotion programme which is less about the provision of facilities and more essentially about training with a high level of face-to-face time of project facilitators with the community. However, providing money for transport is one of the least popular budget items considered by donors investing in many African countries. This may be due to the notorious costs of keeping transport functional, yet this is the single most urgent need to build the capacity of Environmental Health side of the Ministry of Health.

CHCs in Rusizi were unable to fulfill their role because their motorbikes only arrived after the intervention was complete: their fuel allowance *never* reached the district from the headquarters of MoH. By contrast, in Zimbabwe the NGO programme was properly resourced with each of the 6 full-time project officers stationed in the field with motorbikes who were thus each able to supervise 5 CHCs properly, even though none of the EHOs from MoH were mobile. Therefore, although the supervision of CHCs was more expensive in Zimbabwe, it was cost-effective because more beneficiaries could be reached.

By providing motorbikes, a donor is enabling those field officers who are responsible for ensuring safe water sanitation and hygiene throughout the country to be properly mobile. Our research convinces us that if Environmental Health Department of the Ministry of Health was adequately supported to train and monitor CHCs in every village, under 5 deaths would be likely to decrease.

7.4.1 Sustainability of hygiene behaviour change

The main way to assess cost-effectiveness must be the *duration* of the benefits, because if hygiene behaviour back slides and diseases resurge, the intervention has failed to deliver long term sustainability. There are two kinds of sustainability: the behaviour of the individual and the CHC itself. If improving family health, is the main objective, then it is more important that hygiene behaviour changes endure permanently rather than that the CHC, which was purely a conduit of information, survives as a structure. The CHC might not continue as an active group after the initial training, but if hygiene behaviour has changed the individuals within this group permanently, then this is a public health triumph.

We have demonstrated the two main ways that a CHC program can be implemented: either directly by government in a national program supported by NGOs or implemented mainly by NGOs with some government support. Below we show the different advantages and disadvantages to both methods in terms of scaling up.

7.5 Monitoring community

Monitoring people regularly tends to encourage higher levels of behaviour change—people often improve their behaviour even if they receive nothing material as a reward, simply because they know they are being watched (monitored)—the so-called 'Hawthorn Effect'. The institution that should be undertaking this monitoring role (from village to district, through to Provincial and National levels) is, of course, the Ministry of Health, mandated as it is to ensure the public health standards are maintained. Increasing the capacity to monitor is where funding of resources are most needed. Tempting as it is to achieve higher results by more efficiently using NGO supervision (as they are probably more effective in monitoring and implementing WASH programmes) this can never be a long-term solution. If a programme is not sustainable after the NGO has left, then it is not cost-effective. Although the ACF/Africa AHEAD program in Zimbabwe may have been more cost-effective per beneficiary, that programme has 'come and gone', whereas the national CBEHPP under MoH continues to slowly transform every village in Rwanda, going from strength to strength on an upward trend.

7.6 Scaling up the CHC model

Schools are an expected resource in every village, but this was not always the case. A few decades ago, education was recognized as a fundamental human right. Despite the huge challenge, Ministries of Education throughout Africa have almost succeeded in providing schools in most villages and as a result literacy is increasing annually. CHCs provide an informal *adult* education system filling in the gaps that remain in community knowledge and ensuring that communities are health conscious and coordinated to manage their health challenges. Scaling up CHCs to every village takes time, but as there is little infrastructure needed, it is comparatively cost-effective relative to the buildings needed by schools. If Rwanda has been able to coordinate community efforts through CHC in a national structure leading from Village to the President, this can surely be emulated by other countries.

Is scaling up the CHC model possible in those countries that have already missed their MDG targets and are now being challenged to meet the SDGs as well? We suggest that it is indeed possible through three distinct stages: Advocacy, Policy and Program.

- by Regional bodies such as AMCOW advocating at a high level to replicate successful programs across the continent using such declarations as the Kigali Action Plan;

- by ensuring that the CHC model is adopted into policy, so the Ministry of Health can use its existing structures and resources with very little additional cost to organize the Environmental Health Department to start up and monitor CHCs throughout the country;

- by coordinating multiple and diverse efforts by numerous development partners and INGOs into a single national Environmental Health Promotion Program to avoid duplication of efforts and multiplicity of conflicting approaches through a myriad of small NGO projects.

8. Conclusion

The CHC Model 'works'. Community Health Clubs are indeed capable of stimulating public health action cost-effectively. The Model deserves to be replicated in other countries in Africa as soon as possible to alleviate poverty and tackle many preventable diseases in a sustainable, holistic and integrated way. A national Environmental Health program using Community Health Clubs as a vehicle for change in every village, can be reasonably predicted to deliver a wide range of community-led hygiene behavior changes which will ultimately improve family health, social capital and living standards throughout the country. What is badly needed is a clear vision by Governments to adopt the CHC model systematically and invest in building the capacity, not only of the curative wing of Ministry of Health but also the Environmental Health systems which can prevent disease. Countries which adopt the Rwandan approach at national scale are more likely to meet at least Goal 6 of the Sustainable Development Targets by 2030.

Acknowledgements

Both in Rwanda and Zimbabwe the Ministry of Health's Environmental Health Department was a partner in the implantation of the Programme. In Rusizi District of Rwanda, the intervention and monitoring through Ministry of Health in partnership with Africa AHEAD was funded by Bill & Melinda Gates Foundation. In Mberengwa District, Zimbabwe Action Contre la Faim (ACF) in partnership with Zimbabwe AHEAD, funded by the European Commission. We also recognized the contribution of Community Health Club members, their committees and their facilitators who participated in these interventions.

Conflict of interest

The corresponding author was the original designer of the CHC Model and all co-authors have been associated with research or implementation of the CHC program in Rwanda and Zimbabwe, as employees, volunteers or Trustees of Africa AHEAD.

Author details

Juliet Anne Virginia Waterkeyn[1*], Regis Matimati[2], Andrew Muringaniza[2], Agrippa Chigono[2], Amans Ntakarutimana[3], Joseph Katabarwa[4], Zachary Bigirimana[5], Julia Pantoglou[6], Anthony Waterkeyn[1] and Sandy Cairncross[7]

1 Africa AHEAD, South Africa

2 Africa AHEAD, Zimbabwe

3 College of Medicine and Health Sciences, University of Rwanda, Rwanda

4 Africa AHEAD, Tanzania

5 Africa AHEAD, Uganda

6 Institute of Tropical Medicine and International Health, Charité, Germany

7 London School of Hygiene and Tropical Medicine, United Kingdom

*Address all correspondence to: juliet@africaahead.com

IntechOpen

© 2019 The Author(s). Licensee IntechOpen. This chapter is distributed under the terms of the Creative Commons Attribution License (http://creativecommons.org/licenses/by/3.0), which permits unrestricted use, distribution, and reproduction in any medium, provided the original work is properly cited.

References

[1] United Nations. Sustainable Development Goals. 2016. [Internet] Available from: https://www.un.org/sustainabledevelopment/sustainable-development-goals/ [Accessed: 25 October 2015]

[2] United Nations. Millennium Development Report. 2015. [Internet]. Available from: https://www.un.org/millenniumgoals/news.shtml [Accessed: 11 June 2019]

[3] Africa AHEAD Website [Internet] Available from: https://www.africaahead.org/countries/ [Accessed: 30 June 2019]

[4] Waterkeyn J, Cairncross S. Creating a demand for sanitation through community health clubs: A cost-effective intervention in two districts of Zimbabwe. Journal of Social Science and Medicine. 2005;**61**:1958-1970

[5] Mitigation through Community Health Clubs, Manicaland Province, Zimbabwe. Grant No. AID-613-G-12-00001. USAID Report. [Internet]. 2014. Available from: https://www.africaahead.org/wp-content/uploads/2018/11/pa00jtt8.pdf [Accessed: 30 June 2019]

[6] Waterkeyn J. Decreasing communicable diseases through improved hygiene in community health clubs. In: Proceedings of the WEDC Water Engineering & Development Centre Conference. Kampala: Loughborough University; 2005. [Internet] Available from: https://dspace.lboro.ac.uk/dspace-jspui/bitstream/2134/29698/2/WaterkeynJ.pdf [Accessed: 30 June 2019]

[7] Mercy Corps. End of Project Evaluation EC Food Security and Livelihoods Independence Program. 2010. [Internet] Available from: https://www.africaahead.org/sectors/nutrition-sustainable-livelihoods/ [Accessed: 30 July 2019]

[8] Waterkeyn J, Waterkeyn A. Creating a culture of health: Hygiene behaviour change in community health clubs through knowledge and positive peer pressure. Journal of Water, Sanitation and Hygiene for Development. 2013;**3**(2):144-155

[9] Matimati R. Perceptions towards Water, Sanitation and Hygiene among Communities in Chipinge District, Zimbabwe Submitted in Partial Fulfilment of MPH. London: Department of Life Sciences University of Roehampton; 2017. [Internet]. Available from: https://www.africaahead.org/wp-content/uploads/2018/12/Regis-Matimati-Masters-Thesis.pdf [Accessed: 30 June 2019]

[10] Chingono AM. An Investigation on the Impact of the Community Health Clubs Approach on Community Health – Case of Ward 19 in Mberengwa District. Thesis. Zimbabwe. [Internet]: Institute of Water and Sanitation; 2013. Available from: https://www.africaahead.org/wp-content/uploads/2018/12/2013-Agrippa-Thesis-CHC.pdf

[11] Okot P, Waterkeyn J, Kwame V. Rapid sanitation uptake in the internally displaced people camps of northern Uganda through community health clubs. In: Proceedings of the 31st WEDC Water Engineering & Development Centre Conference. Kampala, Uganda: WEDC; 2005. [Internet]. Available from: https://dspace.lboro.ac.uk/dspace-jspui/bitstream/2134/29698/2/WaterkeynJ.pdf [Accessed: 30 June 2019]

[12] Deffner J, Klug T. Participatory implementation of sanitation infrastructure in urban areas of

north-central Namibia. Collaborating Centre for Health Promoting Water Management and Risk Communication University of Bonn - IHPH Institute for Hygiene and Public Health. WHOCC Newsletter No. 21. [Internet]. 2013. Available from: https://africaahead.org/wp-content/uploads/2014/11/2012.Namibia-Water_and_Risk_Vol_21_print.pdf. [Accessed: 25 October 2015]

[13] Maksimsovski N, Waterkeyn A. The Community Health Club Approach in Informal Settlements: Case Study from eThekwini Municipality, Kwa Zulu Natal, South Africa. Durban. South Africa: Water Institute of South Africa; 2010. [Internet]. Available from: https://africaahead.org/wp-content/uploads/2015/08/2010_WISA_eThekwini.pdf [Accessed: 30 June 2019]

[14] Rosenfeld J. Incremental improvements to community water supply systems through community health clubs in the Umzimkhulu local municipality. In: Proceedings of the IWA International Water Association Conference. Addis Ababa, Ethiopia; 2010. [Internet]. Available from https://africaahead.org/wp-content/uploads/2015/08/2010_WISA_-Rosenfeld.pdf [Accessed: 30 June 2019]

[15] Azurduy L, Stakem M, Wright L. Assessment of the Community Health Club Approach: Koinadugu District, Sierra Leone May 12, 2007. International Development Studies. Care International/The Elliott School of International Affairs, The George Washington University; 2007. [Internet]. Available from: https://africaahead.org/wp-content/uploads/2015/08/Capstone-report-on-CHCs.pdf [Accessed: 30 June 2019]

[16] Boone P, Elbourne D, Fazzio I, Fernandes S, Frost C, Jayanty C, et al. Effects of community heath interventions on under 5 mortality in rural Guinea Bissau (EPICS): A cluster-randomised controlled trial. Lancet Glob Health. 2016;**4**:e328-e335. DOI: 10.1016/s2214-109X(16)30048-1

[17] Rosenfeld J. Social Capital and community health clubs in Haiti. PhD Thesis. Gillings School of Public Health, University of North Carolina. 2019. [Internet]. Available from: https://uthscsa-idm-oclc-org.libproxy.uthscsa.edu/docview/2296700336?accountid=7125 [Accessed: 30 September 2019]

[18] Brooks J, Adams A, Bendjemil S, Rosenfeld J. Putting heads and hands together to change knowledge and behaviors: Community health clubs in Port-au-Prince, Haiti. Waterlines. 2015;**34**(4). DOI: 10.3362/1756-3488.2015.033

[19] Lewis K. Community health club and its application for health promotion and community building in Matazano, Guatemala. Journal of Undergraduate Research, 2013-2014. [Internet]. Available from: https://pdfs.semanticscholar.org/cc65/d5626476f0616318f892361676620a4db6ec.pdf [Accessed: 30 June 2019]

[20] Waterkeyn J, Nga N. Low Cost-High Impact: Hygiene Behaviour Change in Vietnam in Community Health Clubs. University of North Carolina – Water Institute Conference; 2011. [Internet]. Available from: http://www.africaahead.com/2017/08/low-cost-high-impact-hygiene-behaviour-change-in-vietnam-in-community-health-clubs/ [Accessed: 30 June 2019]

[21] Ministry of Health Environmental Health Desk. Roadmap for CBEHPP: Community Based Environmental Health Promotion Programme. Rwanda. 2010. [Internet]. Available from: https://www.ircwash.org/sites/default/files/Republic-2010-Roadmap.pdf [Accessed: 30 June 2019]

[22] Government of Rwanda. Economic development and poverty reduction

strategy 2 (EDPRS) 2013-2018. [Internet]. 2018. Available from: http://www.minecofin.gov.rw/fileadmin/templates/documents/NDPR/EDPRS_2.pdf [Accessed: 30 June 2019]

[23] Institute of Policy Analysis and Research (IPAR) - FY 2014/2015/2016 Imihigo Evaluation–Rwanda. http://gasabo.gov.rw/fileadmin/user_upload/Imihigo_evaluation_2014-2015.pdf [Accessed: 12 February 2017]

[24] Kigali Action Plan. African Union 24th Assembly of the Union. 2014;**6**:3.4. [Internet]. [Accessed: 06 June 2019] https://www.africaahead.org/wp-content/uploads/2016/10/20150131_KIGALI-ACTION-PLAN-english-final.pdf

[25] Unicef. Levels & Trends in Child Mortality Report 2014 Estimates Developed by the UN Inter-agency Group for Child Mortality Estimation. 2014. [Internet]. Available from: https://www.who.int/maternal_child_adolescent/documents/levels_trends_child_mortality_2014/en/ [Accessed: 25 October 2015]

[26] Srinavasan L. Tools for Community Participation. A Manual for Training Trainers in Participatory Techniques. New York: PROWESS/United Nations Development Programme; Technical Series Involving Women in Water and Sanitation; 1990

[27] Esrey S, Potash J, Roberts L, et al. Effects of improved water supply and sanitation on ascariasis, diarrhoea, dracunculiasis, hookworm infection, schistosomiasis control: A review. Bulletin of the World Health Organisation. 1991;**69**(5):609-621

[28] Curtis V, Cairncross S. Effect of washing hands with soap on diarrhoea risk in the community: A systematic review. Lancet Infectious Diseases. 2003;**3**(5):275-281

[29] Sinharoy S, Schmidt W-P, Wendt R, Mfura L, Crossett E, Grépin K, et al. Effect of community health clubs on child diarrhoea in western Rwanda: Cluster-randomised controlled trial. Lancet Glob Health. 2017;**5**:e699-e709

[30] Waterkeyn J, Waterkeyn A, Uwingabire F, Pantoglou J, Mbirira M, Ntakarutimana A, et al. The value of monitoring data in an assessment of hygiene behaviour change in Community Health Clubs compared to findings from a cluster Randomised Control Trial in Rwanda. BMC-Public Health – submitted October 2019 [Internet]. Available from: www.africaahead.org/documentation/articles/download_publications/ [Accessed: 30 September 2019]

[31] Sijbesma C, Christoffers T. The value of hygiene promotion: Cost-effectiveness analysis of interventions in developing countries. Health Policy and Planning. 2009;**24**:418-427

[32] Waterkeyn J. Cost Effective Health Promotion: Community Health Clubs. 29th Water Engineering & Development Centre Conference. Abuja, Nigeria. 2003. [Internet]. Available from: https://www.ircwash.org/sites/default/files/Waterkeyn-2003-Cost-effective.pdf [Accessed: 30 June 2019]

[33] Aziz K, Hoque B, Huttly S. Water Supply, Sanitation and Hygiene Education Report of a Health Impact Study in Mirzapur, Bangladesh. Washington. DC: The World Bank. UNDP – World Bank Water and Sanitation Program; 1990

[34] Water Policy. Ministry of Water Resources Development and Management. OFDA Cholera Zimbabwe; 2012. p. 26. [Internet]. Available from: http://ncuwash.org/newfour/wp-content/uploads/2017/08/National-Water-Policy.pdf [Accessed: 30 June 2019]

[35] The Zimbabwe National Sanitation and Hygiene Policy. Zimbabwe. 2012. [Internet]. Available from: http://newfour.ncuwash.org/wp-content/uploads/2017/08/National-Sanitation-and-Hygiene-Policy-Draft-2017.pdf [Accessed: 25 October 2018]

[36] United Nations Human Development Index [Internet]. 2012. Available from: https://en.wikipedia.org/wiki/List_of_countries_by_Human_Development_Index [Accessed: 25 October 2018]

[37] Government of Rwanda. District Development Plan Rusizi District 2013-2018. 2018. Available from: http://www.rusizi.gov.rw/fileadmin/_migrated/content_uploads/DISTRICT_DEVELOPMENT_PLAN_DDP__2013-2018_FINAL.pdf. [Internet]. [Accessed: 30 June 2019]

[38] Government of Rwanda EICV3 District Profile Rusizi. [Internet]. 2011. Available from: www.statistics.gov.rw/file44409/download?token=pPrbUnHM

[39] Waterkeyn J, Mutandiro J. The Community Health Club Approach: Manual for Workshop Participants. Zimbabwe AHEAD. 2009. [Internet]. Available from: https://www.africaahead.org/wp-content/uploads/2019/07/Rural-Zim-Manual-cover.pdf [Accessed: 30 June 2019]

[40] Ministry of Health, Unicef, Africa AHEAD. Gahunda y'abaturage yo Guteza Imbere Ubukikije: Manual for Community Health Club facilitators. Rwanda. 2012. [Internet] Available from: https://www.africaahead.org/documentation/training-tools/rwandan-training-manuals/rwandan-manual-and-toolkit/ [Accessed: 30 June 2019]

[41] Freire P. Education for Critical Consciousness. New York: Seabury; 1973

[42] African Development Bank Group. Water Resource Management, Supply, and Sanitation Zimbabwe. Chapt 7. [Internet]. 2013. Available from http://www.afdb.org/fileadmin/uploads/afdb/Documents/Generic-Documents/9.%20Zimbabwe%20Report_Chapter%207.pdf. [Accessed: 30 June 2019]

[43] Whaley L, Webster J. The effectiveness and sustainability of two demand driven sanitation and hygiene approaches in Zimbabwe. Journal of Water, Sanitation and Hygiene for Development. 2011;**1**(1):20-36

[44] Humphrey JH, Mbuya MNN, Ntozini R. Independent and combined effects of improved water, sanitation, and hygiene, and improved complementary feeding, on child stunting and anaemia in rural Zimbabwe: A cluster-randomised trial. Lancet Glob Health. 2019;7:e132-e147

[45] Pantoglou J. Evaluating Hygiene Behaviour Change within Community Health Clubs in the Rusizi District of Rwanda. Thesis. Berlin: Charité Universitätsmedizin; 2018. [Internet] Available from: https://www.africaahead.org/wp-content/uploads/2018/12/2018.-Pantoglou-Julia-Thesis.pdf [Accessed: 30 June 2019]

[46] Detterman P. Impact Evaluation Report for Gutu and Mberengwa District CHC Programme. Zimbabwe AHEAD; 2012. [Internet] Available from: https://africaahead.org/wp-content/uploads/2015/09/2013.5.Gutu-Mberengwa-Outcome-Evaluation-Report.-PD.pdf [Accessed: 30 June 2019]

[47] Ntakarutimana A, Ekane N. The Performance of Community Health Clubs in Transforming Hygiene Behavior and Sanitation: A Case-Control Study in Kicukiro and Rusizi Districts in Rwanda. Research Development Conference, Stockholm. Sweden. [Internet]. 2017. Available from: https://wedcknowledge.lboro.

ac.uk/resources/conference/40/Ntakarutimana-2798.pdf [Accessed: 06 November 2017]

[48] Ntakirutimana T, Gasana H, Rubuga K. Assessment of Community Based Environmental Health Promotion Program (CBEHPP) achievements and its sustainability in Bugesera District. WaterAid Report. 3rd CBEHPP Workshop. Hotel Umubano, Kigali, Rwanda. May 25th - 26th, 2017. [Internet] Available from: https://www.africaahead.org/wp-content/uploads/2017/05/2016.WaterAid-CBEHPP-Effectiveness.pdf [Accessed: 31 January 2018]

[49] CBEHPP Conference Report "Sharing experience and learning in the implementation of CBEHPP" Hotel Umubano, Kigali, Rwanda. May 25th - 26th, 2017. [Internet] Available from: https://www.africaahead.org/2017/08/3rd-cbehpp-national-workshop/ [Accessed: 29 September 2019]

[50] SNV Annual Report. [Internet]. 2016. p. 25. Available from: http://www.snv.org/public/cms/sites/default/files/explore/download/snv_annual_report_2016_final.pdf [Accessed: 30 June 2019]

Chapter 4

Hygiene Technologies, Water, and Health in the Hellenic World

Stavros Yannopoulos and Asimina Kaiafa-Saropoulou

Abstract

The relation between human health, water, and hygiene facilities has been realized since during the Bronze Age, the explanations of illness and health problems were based on theocratic elements. However, the Greeks during the Classical and mainly the Hellenistic period clearly differentiated their thinking from all other civilizations by inventing philosophy and empirical science. Drains/sewers, baths and toilets, and other sanitary installations are reflecting high cultural and technological level, while they also are associated with observations and ideas about hygiene and medicine. The aim of this paper is to examine the knowledges about the influence of water on human health throughout antiquity. In other words, it focuses on the views that Greeks and Romans had on water quality and its impact on the human body.

Keywords: Asclepieia, Minoan era, Hippocrates, medicine, water quality

1. Introduction

People of Minoan Crete seem to have realized since the third millennium BC that various health problems could be eliminated by well-organized water supply systems and operated sanitation infrastructures. The first known Hellenic philosophical and medical writers, like Thales and Empedocles, also recognized the importance of water for the hygiene and health of people [1].

In many ancient texts, it is mentioned that water quality is considered as a major issue that affected human health. Moreover, water played a major role in the healing process, body relief, and wound care. In the *Iliad* of Homer, for example, Eurypylus asks Patroclus to wash the black blood on his wound with lukewarm water and then put on: "...ἀλλ᾽ ἐμὲ μὲν σὺ σάωσον ἄγων ἐπὶ νῆα μέλαιναν, μηροῦ δ᾽ ἔκταμ᾽ ὀϊστόν, ἀπ᾽ αὐτοῦ δ᾽ αἷμα κελαινὸν/νίζ᾽ ὕδατι λιαρῷ, ἐπὶ δ᾽ ἤπια φάρμακα πάσσε ἐσθλά, τά σε προτί φασιν Ἀχιλλῆος δεδιδάχθαι, ὃν Χείρων ἐδίδαξε δικαιότατος Κενταύρων." This roughly translates as follows: "...But me do thou succour, and lead me to my black ship, and cut the arrow from my thigh, and wash the black blood from it with warm water, and sprinkle thereon kindly healing herbs, whereof men say that thou hast learned from Achilles, whom Cheiron taught, the most righteous of the Centaurs..." (L, 829-831).

Until the sixth and the fifth centuries, health and healing were very much rooted in religion and magic. Furthermore, in the following centuries, till the Roman times, despite the development of philosophy and medical science, those who suffered from various illnesses and pains continued to offer sacrifices, consulted practitioners who prescribed the use of medicinal herbs, or flocked to sanctuaries dedicated to gods associated with healing and health restoring through mysterious ritual a part of which was the presence of water. Within this context the healing god Asclepius, appeared in ancient Greece, and since the sixth century, hundreds of large and small Asclepieia were founded, with common characteristics, providing healthcare facilities. In addition to Asclepius, there have been some other health-related deities, derived from the same family, which were also worshiped at all over the Greek area as well as in Asia Minor, Egypt, or even Rome. According to the Hellenic myth and the Thessalian tradition, Chiron, the wise old centaur, was the fatherly tutor of Asclepius. Chiron's healing activity is certified both by Homer and Pindar. Indeed, due to his knowledge in the medical arts, he is added into the Thessalian healing pantheon. He seems to have possessed healing powers before Asclepius; in fact, he is known as the founder of a family of physicians, who handed down from father to son secrets of the herbs of Pelion and who healed people without payment [2].

Asclepius's skills as a doctor became so advanced, which eventually came to be worshipped as a god of health and disease and was considered to have powers, even to raise the dead, prompting the jealousy of the Olympian gods and the rage of Zeus, who struck him with a lightning bolt. Both his sons, Machaon and Podalirios, and his daughters, Hygeia, Panacea, and Iaso, were also associated with human health. Specifically, Hygeia was the goddess of public health, Panacea was the goddess of therapy, and Iaso was the goddess of cures, remedies, and modes of healing. It is noted that the word hygiene comes from Hygeia the Hellenic goddess of health. Apart from the ca. fourth BC votive relief from Kynouria, where the whole Asclepius' family welcomes a group of supplicants, a unique group of Asclepiads has been found in the complex of Great Baths of Dion. These are six sculptures at least two thirds of the natural size, representing Asclepius and his family, dating back to the early ca. third century AD [3]. There is no doubt that neither the presence of this group of statues nor their location in a complex such Great Baths was selected at random. Their presence indicates the importance of the bath for therapeutic purposes.

In parallel, since the Classical times, the fact that medicine and health practices became more scientific, endeavors provoked a gradual advancement in the design of sanitary and sewerage engineering. Thus, there are many samples of advanced design and construction of lavatories, baths, sewage and drainage systems of those eras, as well as other hygienic structures obviously due to improved understanding of hydraulic and sanitary principles. Later on, Hellenistic period (ca. fourth to first century BC) should be considered as the most progressive time in the design of sanitary and sewerage engineering during antiquity [4]. There is no doubt that many ancient Greek cities in addition with aqueducts and distribution networks were also equipped with advanced drainage systems under their urban grids. That means that the ancients knew that sewerage infrastructures were of equal importance to their cities' water supply systems.

The purpose of this paper is to examine the perceptions of both the people in ancient Greece and Romans about the role and effectiveness of water in healing and generally in human health. In parallel, within the same context and always having in mind the theocratic perceptions of the ancient Greeks, which persist even after the development of medical science in the Classical era, the study traces the role of the gods in relieving human pain and their power to cure ill people through processes in which the element of water had crucial role. In other words, this paper aims to examine the bidirectional connection between the healing powered gods and goddesses and the water springs which they largely determined the location and form of sanctuaries and sanatoriums throughout antiquity.

2. Methodology

Philosophy and all the ideas and theories that ancient Greeks elaborated on the role of the water in human health have been the real basis for the development of hygiene technology from antiquity till nowadays.

Extensive drainage and sewerage systems and elaborate sanitary infrastructures, such as baths and flushing toilets, were in use since prehistoric in cases where settlements had urban organization and central authority, like those of Minoan Crete and other Aegean islands. Influenced by the progress of philosophy of Classical and Hellenistic periods on public health and especially in the provision of saving drinking water and adequate sewage disposal, Greeks advanced sanitary engineering through antiquity by constructing sanitary infrastructures and hygiene facilities or creating new ones. Romans having in mind the past technology and hygienic practices of the Greeks, they advanced the known sanitary techniques by implementing extensive systems for public and private hygiene, which formed the basis of modern sanitary technology.

In order to review the role of water in sanitation and preservation of the public health, antiquity texts from ancient Greek and Roman literature have been gathered, related to philosophy, medicine, architecture, and poetry. In parallel, many archeological evidences from all over Greece have been gathered and recorded for the same purpose.

As it was impossible to quote all the texts related to this issue, the most characteristics of them have been chosen and cited that means the ones that express and prove better the conditions and practices through which ancient Greeks and Romans are conductive to maintaining health, prevention, or healing diseases through cleanliness.

3. Prehistory

The first Minoan settlements were established in dry- and water-scarce sites, where the Minoans developed an advanced, comfortable, and hygienic lifestyle, as manifested by water supply systems, flushing lavatories, public and private baths, and very effective sewers and drains. All Minoan palaces have been found to have high-quality hygienic facilities, water dispensers with running water, and an underground drainage system. Besides, Minoan religion required believers to be always clean. Sacred fountains, lustral basins for ritual bathing, and other purgatory facilities were found in several palaces, cities, and other Minoan settlements next to domestic rooms or near the entrances [4].

The presence of such sophisticated hygiene and body care infrastructures must be very much connected with high-level medicine and very well-evolved healing methods. However, despite the fact that grooming and physical hygiene are depicted in many wall paintings, there are no frescoes at all that give any information about medicine and physician processes. Similarly, none of the numerous Linear B clay tablets provide any such information, although the word doctors are mentioned in their text.

4. Archaic till Hellenistic times

4.1 Water quality and human health

The effectiveness of water on the human body was particularly concerned within the ancient world. Numerous ancient written sources, concerning water and hygiene, confirmed that water had beneficial or harmful effects on human health and played a crucial role in the body or mental healing, depending on its quality; in other words it defined in many ways the art of medicine. What is even more interesting is the connection of water presence with theocratic concepts, superstitions, and processes in sacred complexes dedicated to gods with healing powers. Plutarch

(*Αιτίαι Φυσικαί*), Vitruvius (*De Architectura*), Pliny (*Naturalis Historiae*), and Aristotle (*Problems*) express similar views on the effect of water quality on human health [5, 6]. Alcmaeon of Croton, in the first half of the fifth century, was the first who mentioned that the health of people are very much connected to the quality of water (Aetius, V, 30, 1), which, according to Vitruvius (*De Architectura* I, 4, 9, 10), was examined by the senses, taste, smell, appearance, and temperature. Tasteless, cool, odorless, and colorless water was considered as the best, in contrary to stagnant and marshy waters that are inappropriate resulting in various diseases.

Aristotle, who mentions the difference between drinking water and that which was used for all other daily needs in his *Politics* (1330b), believed in the importance of water in the human body and underlined that water causes more diseases than food, since food contains water (*Problems* I, 13, 14, 861a) ([1], p. 51). Hippocrates and Vitruvius make extensive reports to diseases which were caused by poor-quality water. The contribution of water to the physical and mental development of humans, in addition to clean air, is also underlined by Diodorus of Sicily, who claims that water "*...πρός ὑγείαν σωμάτων καί ῥώμην συμβάλλεται...*" ("*water...also contribute to the health and vigour of their bodies...*"). Many ancient writers pointed the fact that the Athenians were affable and had a loud voice and great memory due to the excellent quality of water that flowed in their town from Hymettus, Penteli, and Parnitha. Diodorus of Sicily also emphasizes the contribution of water in physical and mental health along with fresh air (*...πρός ὑγείαν σωμάτων καί ῥώμην συμβάλλεται...*).

According to the ancient people of the Greek area, the quality of water depended on the geological profile of the spot from which it flowed. Moreover, the orientation of springs and their position in relation to the direction of the winds are also largely related to the water quality of an area which affects public health. Athenaeus, for example, referring to Hippocrates, records the primacy of the waters that are eastbound and are exposed to the eastern winds. He believes that those waters are "λαμπρά, *εὐώδη καί κοῦφα*" ("*...One should, however, ... drink water which is light and transparent in appearance, light, too, in actual weight and free from solid matter...*"). The most harmful waters of the human body were marshes. The ancients knew that swamps, marshlands, and, generally, naturally occurring collections of stagnant water could cause dangerous or even mortal diseases, such as malaria. Marshes at the edge of Loudias lake/river next to the capital city of Macedonia, Pella, affected badly the public health so much that people there both had "*...a spleen twice as large as (their) belly...*" ("*τῆς κοιλίας τόν σπλῆν' ἔχοντα διπλάσιον," Athenaeus, Deipnosofistai A, 348e-f*) and their "...faces pale..." ("*ἐτύγχανον ... χλωροί ὄντες," Athenaeus, Deipnosofistai A, 352a*) which both of them are malaria symptoms. Moreover, the inhabitants of Troizina, which were drinking inappropriate water, had also health problems especially on their feet. Athenaeus also dealt extensively with the quality of water in various parts of the world and many times repeats information written years ago. Among others, he mentioned that the Nile water was very fertilizing and fresh. Hence, it loosens the bowels and aids digestion, since it contains a soda ingredient (*Deipnosofistai* B, 41). On the other hand, he attributed the death of many Egyptians to the Nile water, when sometimes droughts had occurred in the Nile valley and the flow of water became poisonous for humans.

Hippocrates since the end of the fifth century BC developed a medical approach, which was based on observation of clinical signs and rational conclusions and not to the religions or magical beliefs, or to the displeasure of the gods, or other supernatural causes [6, 7]. Specifically, for the first time, he supported the rationality of the etiology of disease and separated real medicine from religious superstitions. He applied logic so as to understand various diseases and find ways to cure them. In his texts he often mentions the effect of drinking water on the human body. He attributes the appearance of some diseases or even the weakness of some people to the bad water quality, of high salinity, that means salty, bitter, nitrite, sulfate, ferrous, acidic waters, or even rain waters which are perishable and can damage human cells or irritate the skin. Hippocrates pointed out that the quality of rainwater is rapidly getting worse with strange smell and unpleasant taste. Drinking it without pre-boiling or pre-filtering it, can provoke damages in human cells by causing stomach aches, poisoning, and vomiting. In addition, especially the water, which falls after a long period of drought, is similarly dangerous for human health, since it is essentially derived from a dirty atmosphere (*Περί Αέρων, Υδάτων, Τόπων*, and *Περί Χυμών*). Thus, other waters affect human health negatively or cause even death, even though they are appropriate in other cases. Hippocrates mentions that seawater is certainly not drinkable; however, a sea bath could be beneficial in healing skin irritation or wounds (*Περί υγρών χρήσιος*).

Contamination of water that used to run through lead supply pipes was a very serious issue of the Roman era concerning public health. Vitruvius theorized about the impact of lead erosion on water quality, which affects badly the human health, and recommended the use of clay pipelines where the water preserves its good taste; therefore, it is appropriate for drinking: "*...etiamque multo salubrior est ex tubules aqua quam per fistulas quod plumbum videtur esse ideo vitiosum, quod ex eo cerussa nscitur. Haec autem dicitur esse nocens corporibus humanis. Ita quod ex eo procreatur, 'si' id est vitiosum, non est dubium, quin ipsum quoque non sit salubre. Exemplar autem ab artificibus plumbariis possumus accipere, quod palloribus occupatos habent corporis colores. Namque cum fundendo plumbum flatur, vapor ex eo insidens corporis artus et in diem exurens eripit ex membris eorum sanguinis virtutes. Itaque minime fistulis plumbeis aqua duci videtur, si volumus eam habere salubrem.*" This roughly translates as follows: "...Water conducted through earthen pipes is more wholesome than that through lead; indeed that conveyed in lead must be injurious, because from it white lead is obtained, and this is said to be injurious to the human system. Hence, if what is generated from it is pernicious, there can be no doubt that itself cannot be a wholesome body. This may be verified by observing the workers in lead, who are of a pallid colour; for in casting lead, the fumes from it fixing on the different members, and daily burning them, destroy the vigour of the blood; water should therefore on no account be conducted in leaden pipes if we are desirous that it should be wholesome. That the flavour of that conveyed in earthen pipes is better, is shewn at our daily meals, for all those whose tables are furnished with silver vessels, nevertheless use those made of earth, from the purity of the flavour being preserved in them..." (De Architectura 8, 6, 10-11).

Opinions on this issue conflict. For example, Hodge [8] excludes the possibility of poisoning or even of the bad impact on the health of Roman citizens, in the long run, from the lead water pipes [9] because, on the one hand, the continuous flow of water into them does not allow the taking of harmful substances at least to such an extent as to affect public health, and solidified calcium deposits on the inner walls of the pipes after a period of continuous use were acted insulating, preventing any contact of the water with the lead. On the contrary, Kobert, accepting the remarks of Vitruvius, made the firm declaration that the ancients had to suffer from poisoning from lead water pipes [9]. Other scholars, professing themselves, note that lead poisoning was commonplace and sometimes it was taking epidemic proportions [10, 11].

Given these, ancient physician's tried to find ways to improve the quality of water that should be swallowed so as to protect the population from waterborne diseases [1]. Both the ancient Greeks and Romans were aware of various ways to control and upgrade water quality so as to avoid many illnesses that were caused by drinking contaminated water. Many different water purifying methods are mentioned in ancient texts written by Vitruvius, Hippocrates, Athenaeus, or Galen, which include the boiling of water over the fire, heating of water under the sun, dipping of heated iron into the water, and filtrating through gravel and sand. Hippocrates discovered many of the healing powers of water. He invented the practice of sieving water and obtained a bag-type filter, known as "Hippocratic sleeve," the main purpose of which was to trap sediments that caused bad tastes or odors. Boiling water must be the most common treatment of water cleaning. Athenaeus copied an information from Herodotus' *Histories* who had mentioned that the king of Persia always took with him a drinking water, which comes from Choaspes springs, from Susa. This was the only water he used to drink. This water had been boiled and then was transferred to silver jars in four-wheeled wagons, following the king. Ctesias of Cnidus certified that the water was boiled and then placed in the cans for use and added that it was very light and enjoyable. Athenians, on the other hand, since the fifth century BC used to mix a part of wine with nine parts of water. Chemical compounds that are produced in the mixture have the power to destroy the germs that cause diseases such as typhoid, dysentery, salmonella, or even cholera [12].

4.2 Water in medicine and its role in healing process

The roots of modern medicine could be traced in the late Archaic and Classical Greece [6]. Even though medical history goes back to Homeric times, illnesses were regarded as a punishment and healing as a gift from the gods. Classical and Hellenistic eras are also very important as far as the evolution in sanitation and hygiene technology in the Hellenic world matters. That is undoubtedly related to the scientific approach to the illnesses and the study of medicine, which never completely disconnected from various religious approaches or from sanctuaries related to health and cure, such as the Asclepieia, which were transformed somehow to medical schools and hospitals. During this period there were two different approaches in Hellenic medicine: (a) the religious medicine of god Asclepius and (b) the philosophical medicine of Hippocrates, Herophilus, Erasistratus, and Asclepiades.

Quite early ancient Greeks transferred medical powers from Mount Olympus down to earth. Thus, appeared Asclepius. Galen, who believed in the myths, remarks that before Asclepius medicine was based on experience and people were healed using only plants, while he made it an empirical science, by introducing new and different methods of healing. Accordingly, to the Hellenic mythology, Asclepius was the son of Coronis and Apollo, who carried him to the centaur Chiron. He raised Asclepius and instructed him in the art of medicine. Besides, according to an etymological approach, the compound name Ασκληπιός (Asclepius) consists of the Hellenic words ασκείν (practicing) and ήπιος (mild), meaning the one that gently removes pain and illness. Another etymological analysis the Hellenic word Asclepius derives from the Hellenic verb σκελλώ (do something hard) which, along with the privative phoneme A and the word ήπιos (mild), implies the one who prevents drying and necrosis of the body gently, with medicine [13, 14].

Specifically, Asclepius was a popular and influential healing figure throughout the Mediterranean [15]. He also became so popular across Greece for his extraordinary healing skills that he was worshipped everywhere in the ancient Hellenic world and its colonies. The healer and comforting god was much loved in the entire Greece. In the south his cult was officially swept at least since the end of sixth century BC, even though his activities and contribution to the art of medicine were widely known since Homer, which is ca. eighth century BC [13, 16–18]. In the north the first established archeological evidences for the worship of Asclepius go back at least the first half of the ca. fourth century BC, which are mainly coming from the colonies, for example, from Amphipolis, Olynthus, and Potidaea [19].

There were sanctuaries located in remote but beautiful areas, well-known as Asclepieia or Asclepieions, dedicated to the healer god, which functioned as centers of medical advice, prognosis, and healing. More than 300 *Asclepieia* existed across the ancient Hellenic world. They swept over Greece during ca. fifth century BC. Since then, the cult of the healer god has become increasingly popular. That means that almost every Hellenic city had an *Asclepieion*, which means a sanctuary dedicated to the health of citizens through the worship of the healer god [13, 16–18].

The geomorphology and the natural environment were playing an important role in the choice of the location of Asclepius' sanctuaries, as they were facilitating the development of worship. In each case, rich aquifers and natural springs were a major factor for the operation of these sanctuaries. In addition, the presence of rivers or constantly flowing torrents was composing an ideal environment for sacred centers dedicated to Asclepius. Apart from this environment profile, every sanctuary had three basic characteristics connected to water, fountains, hygiene facilities, and baths. After all there was a close relationship between thermal springs, Asclepius, and medicine [16, 18, 20].

They were not the only areas of worship but also medical care centers. Thousands of people used to visit them to be healed from various problems and physical or mental health illnesses. They were combining experimental therapeutic methods with various religions and magical elements and the healing power of water. These included sacrifices, prayers, proper nutrition, taking of medicinal plants, hearing theatrical and musical performances, and finally hypnotherapy. Special procedures, such as catharsis, exercises, massage, and fasting, were taking place there in order to obtain physical and mental recreation and healing. For those buildings such as theaters, gymnasia, hippodromes, and sanitation installations were constructed next to the central temple or to the main buildings of every sanctuary, where physicians were practicing medicine. Finally, the crucial role of water in the procedures or sacred rituals and ceremonies in every Asclepieion is associated with the existence of fountains, springs, and baths. Fountains were perhaps the most basic element of Asclepius' sanctuaries, as the supply of running water was essential not only for ritual ceremonies but also for all of the healing practices which were carried out there. Usually, the required water for purifications and other religious and therapeutic procedures was drawn from tanks, fountains, or sources that were embedded in the sanctuary. It is worth mentioning that a water source constituted an indispensable feature in the sanctuaries of Asclepius [13, 17, 18]. In the temple of Asclepieion of Corinth, the necessary water for the cult and hygiene was drawn from Lerna spring. It was located in the southern site of Lerna court beneath the avaton and was praised as "...the sweetest..." ("...ἥδιστον...") (Athenaeus, Deipnosofistai D, 156). The Asclepieion was a place where people were coming to be healed of their diseases. The complex included dining rooms, bathing facilities, dormitories, and other structures.

In Athens the fountain was built above the spring. It was incorporated in the avaton of Asclepius temple and had a circular form, just like the natural carving on the rock of the Acropolis' hill from where the water was outflowing [21]. A fountain has been also found in the Asclepieion of Kos [20], while the natural water source in the sanctuary of Asclepius at Levina in Crete has been also molded in fountain [22, 23]. Furthermore, an inscription of ca. second century BC from Veroia informs the existence of a big, complicated fountain with many spouts in the Asclepieion of the city [24].

The worship of Asclepius was often inserted to already existing sanctuaries of deities who were related to his origin and life, like his father Apollo, or were having similar curative powers [13, 25]. The coexistence of Asclepius, Apollo, Hygeia, and occasionally goddesses Artemis and Demeter was also equally common [13, 17, 26].

In Afytos of Chalkidiki, the cult of Asclepius coexisted with the sanctuary of Zeus Ammon. The relation of Zeus with water and healing is not disputed so as the appropriateness of the area which was of great natural beauty and had rich vegetation, plus water abundance. The baths, built in ca. second century BC nearby, were undoubtedly associated with the healer god, as various findings indicate the practice of medical art in some of the rooms [27]. Often Asclepius was worshiped in areas which were also dedicated to the cult of Nymphs [17, 20], probably due to the common natural environment that these deities were required. Along with the cult of Asclepius in Lebena existed the worship of Hermes, Nymphs, and river Acheloos [22].

Besides Asclepius who was widely known as a healer god, in Macedonia similar properties seem to attribute to *Darron* (in Hellenic Δάρρων). According to Hesychius, *Darron* was a *Macedonian demon to whom they pray for the healing of sick people* (*Μακεδονικὸς δαίμων, ᾧ ὑπὲρ τῶν νοσούντων εὔχονται*). According to another opinion, the name *Δάρρων* (*Darron*) is another form of the name *Θάρρων ή Θάρσων*, which means courage, which is accompanying the first name of a healer god, Apollo or Asclepius, meaning that he gives courage to patients and helps in their health recovery [28]. Recently a sanctuary has been found in Pella, which is related with an inscription to the worship of demon Darron. Several findings plus architectural remains, such as a purification of a cistern, a well, a fountain, a sink near the entrance, are similar to those found in places dedicated to Asclepius. Possibly *Darron* was a local, demonic being with therapeutic attributes, perhaps attendant of Asclepius, like Telesphoros, worshiped by the Macedonians probably together with Asclepius or Health [29].

Both Pliny and Vitruvius tried to mention all the benefits from therapeutic baths and the use of water, which were also pointed out by Homer, ages ago: "...ἡ δὲ τετάρτη ὕδωρ ἐφόρει καὶ πῦρ ἀνέκαιε πολλὸν ὑπὸ τρίποδι μεγάλῳ· ἰαίνετο δ' ὕδωρ. αὐτὰρ ἐπεὶ δὴ ζέσσεν ὕδωρ ἐνὶ ἤνοπι χαλκῷ, ἕς ῥ' ἀσάμινθον ἕσασα λό' ἐκ τρίποδος μεγάλοιο, θυμῆρες κεράσασα, κατὰ κρατός τε καὶ ὤμων, ὄφρα μοι ἐκ κάματον θυμοφθόρον εἵλετο γυίων..." (κ360). This roughly translates as follows: "... But when the water boiled in the bright bronze, she set me in a bath, and bathed me with water from out the great cauldron, mixing it to my liking, and pouring it over my head and shoulders, till she took from my limbs soul-consuming weariness..." It was well-known that hydrotherapy is beneficial for muscle aches, daily stress, illnesses, or injuries. The heated water relaxes, improves body circulation, and reduces inflammation.

As for Hippocrates, the therapeutic bath is a medical procedure and should be taken under detailed instructions (diet and regimen in acute diseases 65): "...The bath is useful in many diseases, in some of them when used steadily, and in others when not so. ... And if the patient be not bathed properly, he may be thereby hurt in no inconsiderable degree, for there is required a place to cover him that is free of smoke, abundance of water, materials for frequent baths, but not very large, unless this should be required. It is better that no friction should be applied, but if so, a hot soap (smegma) must be used in greater abundance than is common, and an affusion of a considerable quantity of water is to be made at the same time and afterwards repeated... But the person who takes the bath should be orderly and reserved in his manner, should do nothing for himself, but others should pour the water upon him and rub him, and plenty of water, of various temperatures, should be in readiness for the douche, and the affusions quickly made; and sponges should be used instead of the strigil, and the body should be anointed when not quite dry. ... and a man should not be washed immediately after gruel or drink; ... In general, it (bath) suits better with cases of pneumonia than in ardent fevers; for the bath soothes the pain in the side, chest, and back; concocts the sputa, promotes expectoration, improves the respiration, and allays lassitude; for it soothes the joints and outer skin, and is diuretic, removes heaviness of the head, and moistens the nose. Such are the benefits to be derived from the bath, if all the proper requisites be present; but if one or more of these be wanting, the bath, instead of doing good, may rather prove injurious ... it is by no means a suitable thing in these diseases to persons whose bowels are too loose, or when they are unusually confined, and there has been no previous evacuation; neither must we bathe those who are debilitated, nor such as have nausea or vomiting, or bilious eructations; nor such as have hemorrhage from the nose, unless it is less than required at that stage of the disease (with those stages you are acquainted), but if the discharge be less than proper, one should use the bath, whether in order to benefit the whole body or the head alone. If then the proper requisites are at hand, and the patient is well disposed to the bath, it may be administered once every day, or if the patient is fond of the bath there will be no harm, though he should take it twice in the day...".

Among others, they recognized various types of hot and medicinal springs whose sulfurous waters refresh the human body. Pliny in *Naturalis Historia* tried to refer the powerful properties of water for humans, which are so numerous that no one could ever describe: "... *quapropter ante omnia ipsarum potentiae exempla ponemus. cunctas enim enumerare quis mortalium queat*?" (*Naturalis Historia* 31, 1-8). This roughly translates as follows: "...*It will be only proper, therefore, in the first place to set forth some instances of the powerful properties displayed by this element; for as to the whole of them, what living mortal could describe them?...*" He mentioned the presence of different kinds of waters springing forth from specific spots, cold or hot or even tepid with positive influence on human health, in fact curative for specific diseases: "...*alibi tepidae, egelidae, atque auxilia morborum profitentes et e cunctis animalibus hominum tantum causa erumpentes augent numerum deorum nominibus variis urbesque condunt...*" This roughly translates as follows: "... Then, again, there are others that are tepid only, or lukewarm, announcing thereby the resources they afford for the treatment of diseases, and bursting forth, for the benefit of man alone, out of so many animated beings...," "......*vaporant et in mari fuere, mediosque inter fluctus existit aliquid valetudini salutare...*" This roughly translates as follows: "......*There are others, too, which send forth their vapours in the sea even, thus providing resources for the health of man in the very midst of the waves...*", "...*Iam generatim nervis prosunt pedibusve aut coxendicibus, aliae luxatis fractisve, inaniunt alvos, sanant vulnera, capiti, auribus privatim medentur, oculis vero Ciceronianae...*" This roughly translates as follows: "...*According to their respective kinds, these waters are beneficial for diseases of the sinews, feet, or hips, for sprains or for fractures; they act, also, as purgatives upon the bowels, heal wounds, and are singularly useful for affections of the head and ears: indeed, the waters of Cicero are good for the eyes...*", "...*In Campania, too, are the waters of Sinuessa, remedial, it is said, for sterility in females, and curative of insanity in men...*", "... *in Aenaria insula calculosis mederi...... idem contingit in Velino lacu potantibus...*" This roughly translates as follows: "*The waters of the island of Ænaria are curative of urinary calculi,*[1] *it is said...... Patients suffering from these complaints may be cured also by drinking the waters of Lake Velia...*", "...*iuxta Romam Albulae aquae volneribus medentur, egelidae hae, sed Cutiliae in Sabinis...prope morsus videri possit, aptissimae stomacho, nervis, universo corpori...*" This roughly translates as follows: "... *The tepid waters of Albula,*[1] *near Rome, have a healing effect upon wounds. Those of Cutilia, in the Sabine territory...seem to be the best situation for stomach ailment, on the whole body...*".

5. Roman era

Along with the Greeks, the Etruscans, the people who lived in the area south of the Arno River, had linked individual hygiene and public health with the presence of clean water but with the immediate removal of dirt and excess water from very early. That's why they had developed the hydraulic art and had built plumbing facilities from very early, sophisticated, so that they were used as models by the Romans. Even Cloaca maxima in Rome was built by Etruscan engineers around 600 BC, while the first aqueduct in Rome in 312 BC is also attributed to them [30]. Also, the thermal baths of Etruria (Chianciano, Del Sasso), as well as the famous centers of Etruscan medicine, have been of a magical religious character.

Roman medicine, very much like Greek medicine, in parallel with its scientific base, was very strongly connected with religious influences and superstitions [6]. However, apart from a large number of doctors and physicians who developed the science and practice of medicine, the Romans' real contributions to healthcare are the hygiene and sanitation technologies, water sophisticated supply, and sewage systems. Hygiene in Roman era included baths and toilets in private and public buildings. The Romans developed the art of baths, which in every case had as an essential condition to the adequate supply of water and the presence of an efficient drainage system. Many of the baths were grandiose bands that operated until sunset and were open for the sick up to 2 hours and in the afternoon for the rest of the guests.

In addition to the baths, the Romans greatly promoted the use of natural hot springs scattered throughout the Empire [31]. Most of them had healing properties and could relieve various body or even insane sufferings. The fact that therapeutic bathing in medicinal and thermal springs provide relief for many complaints was very well-known since the Hellenistic period; nevertheless the Romans were the ones who developed systematically [32]. High-temperature springs were treated as a special kind of waters ages before the Roman era. In fact, some of them were considered to be sacred, with supernatural powers and special healing properties. In ancient Greek and Latin literature numerous well known thermal springs were reported. Many of them seemed to have components which give them different properties, and make them suitable for the treatment of different diseases.

The Romans built splendid baths on the sites of hot springs in all over the empire, where many people flocked in order to find healing or relief for their illness. This practice of them was certainly not free from their theocratic perceptions. Besides, Vitruvius recommended spots with natural water springs as the best choice for shrines dedicated to every god or goddess, especially to those connected to healing: "*...naturalis autem decor sic erit, si imum omnibus templis saluberrimae regiones aquarumque fontes in iis locis idonei eligentur in quibus fana constituantur, deinde maxime Aesculapio Saluti, quorum deorum plurimi medicinis aegri curari videntur. cum enim ex pestilenti in salubrem locum corpora aegra translata fuerint et e fontibus salubribus aquarum usus subministrabuntur, celerius convalescent...*" (*De Architectura, 1, 2, 7*). This roughly translates as follows: "*......Natural consistency arises from the choice of such situations for temples as possess the advantages of salubrious air and water; more especially in the case of temples erected to Æsculapius, to the Goddess of Health, and such other divinities as possessing the power of curing diseases. For thus the sick, changing the unwholesome air and water to which they have been accustomed to those that are healthy, sooner convalesce; and a reliance upon the divinity will be therefore increased by proper choice of situation...*".

Ages later, Caelius Aurelianus, a Roman citizen who lived in the fifth century AD in the town Sicca in the African province Numidia, supported the therapeutic use of sea bathing as a very relieving and curative body treatment. He suggested people to lay in a bathtub full of hot ocean water the high temperature of which may maintain by dipping in flaming iron bars.

In the second century AD Galen, who linked healthcare with diet, use of water baths, and hygiene [30], did not consider at length with the benefits of bathing and spring waters. His medical references include the beneficial use of the thermomineral waters [32, 33], while he recommended the additional use of baths not by using hot waters. The water should be neither tepid nor icy, as it strengthens the whole body and makes the skin thick and tough [34].

Moreover, Pedanius Dioscorides, a Greek physician of the first century AD, suggested that a mixture of an equal measure of water and must (grape pulp) boiled over a soft fire until the water is used up has laxative effects for the human body. Talking about herbal medicine in his five-volume book *De Materia Medica* (5, 13), he also mentioned that for the same purposes, someone can mix an equal amount of sea water, rainwater, honey, and must, pour it out into another jar, and set it in the sun for 40 days.

6. Conclusions

The connection between public health, clean water, and sanitation has been explored since antiquity. Medicine in Classical and Hellenistic times became gradually more based on clinical observations and scientific investigations. Before that time advances, medicine was entirely confined to religious beliefs and rituals [35]. Since the sixth century BC, philosophy began to flourish in the Greek cities of the Aegean and the Ionian coast of Asia Minor. The environment was mature enough, and scientific medicine was enabled to be born. Physicians attempted to identify material causes for illnesses; in parallel, people never stopped flocking to sanctuaries so as to find succor for their illnesses. They usually preferred Asclepieia, which were located in areas with lush vegetation, rich, and fresh water.

Ancient authors many times commented about the influence of different kinds of water on people's health. Thus, they were all aware that waterborne infections have been among the main causes of people's deaths. The Romans believed that illnesses had a cause and that the bad health is connected to bad water and sewage. Both Greek and Romans were trying to improve the quality of water using settling tanks, filters, or boiling it, which was the most recommended of all existing methods.

Influenced by the advent and progress of philosophy in Classical and Hellenistic periods, sanitation and hygienic conditions and especially medicine became gradually more based on clinical observations and scientific investigations.

The role of water is crucial in the Hippocratic medicine. Specifically, what is shown here is that diseases are less frequent in cities with an eastern aspect, since the waters, which flow there, is considered to be healthier and more suitable for drinking.

In conclusion, although the above descriptions do not provide a complete picture of urban sanitation technologies in ancient Greece, they serve to illustrate the fact that such technologies were in use in ancient Greece since about 4000 years ago. These advanced technologies, developed originally in Minoan era, were subsequently transferred to the Mycenaean civilization and then the Archaic, Classical, and Hellenistic Greece. These sanitation and hygienic technologies were further improved during the Roman period formed, for example, a type of lavatory which survived with limited modifications for more than 1500 years. Based on historical and archeological evidences, the present-day progress in urban water technology as well as in comfortable and hygienic living is clearly not a recent development. The Greeks considered pioneers in developing the basic sanitation technologies in the western world. They placed emphasis on providing an urban hygienic environment, with emphasis in a sustainable way since the prehistoric times.

Undoubtedly ancient Hellenic and Roman views contain excellent remarks on the role of the water and hygiene with regard to people's health. For that many of which have survived until modern times. Centuries later, in the late nineteenth century, the role of personal and public hygiene and water on people's health was really very well understood. The fact that hygiene technologies and safe drinking water are intimately tied to human health has been so perfectly conceivable that Lewis Thomas mentioned [36]: The connection between public health, clean water and sanitation has been explored since antiquity. Medicine in Classical and Hellenistic times became gradually more based on clinical observations and scientific investigations. Before that time advances, medicine was entirely confined to religious beliefs and rituals [35]. Since the sixth century BC, philosophy began to flourish in the Greek cities of the Aegean and the Ionian coast of Asia Minor. The environment was mature enough, and scientific medicine was enabled to be born. Physicians attempted to identify material causes for illnesses. In parallel, people never stopped flocking to sanctuaries so as to find succor for their illnesses. In the late Hellenistic period, the knowledge of the ancient world of hygienic matter was incorporated in legislative rules.

Ancient authors many times commented about the influence of different kinds of water on people's health. Thus, they were all aware that waterborne infections have been among the main causes of people's deaths. There is no question that our health has improved spectacularly in the past century. One thing seems certain: It did not happen because of improvements in medicine, or medical science, or even the presence of doctors, much of the credit should go to the plumbers and sanitary engineers of the western world [37].

Author details

Stavros Yannopoulos[1] and Asimina Kaiafa-Saropoulou[2*]

1 Faculty of Engineering, School of Rural and Surveying Engineering, Aristotle University of Thessaloniki, Thessaloniki, Greece

2 School of Architecture, Aristotle University, Thessaloniki, Greece

*Address all correspondence to: minakasar@gmail.com

IntechOpen

© 2019 The Author(s). Licensee IntechOpen. This chapter is distributed under the terms of the Creative Commons Attribution License (http://creativecommons.org/licenses/by/3.0), which permits unrestricted use, distribution, and reproduction in any medium, provided the original work is properly cited. (cc) BY

References

[1] Vuorinen HS, Juuti PS, Katko TS. History of water and health from ancient civilizations to modern times. Water Science and Technology: Water Supply. 2007;7(1):49-57

[2] Gorrini ME. Healing heroes in Thessaly: Chiron the Centaur. In: The Archaeological Work of Thessaly and Sterea Greece, Proceedings of the 1st Archaeological Symposium; 27 February 2003 to 2 March 2003; Volos, Greece; 2003. pp. 283-295

[3] El-Esawi MA. Nonzygotic embryogenesis for plant development. In: Anis M, Ahmad N, editors. Plant Tissue Culture: Propagation, Conservation and Crop Improvement. Singapore: Springer; 2016. pp. 583-598

[4] Pandermalis D. Dion. Archaeology. 1989;**33**:29-34 (in Hellenic)

[5] Yannopoulos S, Yapijakis C, Kaiafa-Saropoulou A, Antoniou G, Angelakis A. History of sanitation and hygiene technologies in the Hellenic world. Water, Sanitation and Hygiene for Development. 2017;7(2):163-180

[6] Kaiafa A. Water and sanitation systems in the Hellenistic and Roman periods in Macedonia [thesis]. Aristotle University of Thessaloniki, Greece; 2008 (in Hellenic)

[7] Cilliers L, Retief FP. Medical practice in Graeco-Roman antiquity. Curationis. 2006;**29**(2):34-40

[8] Yapijakis C. Hippocrates of Kos, the Father of Clinical Medicine, and Asclepiades of Bithynia, the Father of Molecular Medicine. Review in Vivo. 2009;**23**:507-514

[9] Hodge T. Vitruvius, lead pipes and lead poisoning. American Journal of Archaeology. 1981;**85**(4):486-491

[10] Kobert R. Chronische Bleivergiftung im Klassische Altertum. In: Diergard P, editor. Beiträge aus der Geschichte der Chemie dem Gedächtnis von Georg W.A. Kahlbaum. Leipzig and Vienna: Deuticke; 1909. pp. 103-109

[11] Waldron H. Lead poisoning in the ancient world. Medical History. 1973;**17**:392-399

[12] Mackie A, Townshend A, Waldron H. Lead concentration in bones from Roman York. Journal of Archaeological Science. 1975;**2**:235-237

[13] Chadjivasileiou V. The medical properties of wine according to Hippocrates. The wines of Kos, Χάρις Χαίρε, Studies in memory of Charis Kantzia, A, 269-275, Athens; 2004 (in Greek)

[14] Edelstein EJ, Edelstein L. Asclepius: A Collection and Interpretation of the Testimonies. Baltimore, USA: The Johns Hopkins University Press; 1945

[15] Holtzman B. Asklepios. In: Lexicon Iconographicum Mythologiae Classicae II. Zürich—München, Germany; 1986. pp. 863-897

[16] Morehouse LR. Dismemberment and devotion: Anatomical votive dedication in Italian popular religion. Honors Projects. Paper 17; 2012. Available at: http://digitalcommons.macalester.edu/classics_honors/17/ [Accessed: 10 March 2015].

[17] Kerenyi K. Der Göttliche Arzt: Studien über Asklepios und seine Kultstätten. Basel, Switzerland: Ciba Aktiengesellschaft; 1948. 121 p

[18] Martin R, Metzger H. La religion grecque. Presses Universitaires de France. Coll. "Sup-L' Historien" 22. Paris, France; 1976. 208 p

[19] Kallegia A. Asclepieia, ancient health centers. Corpus. 2000;**19**:60-72 (in Hellenic)

[20] Comella A. I rilievi votive greci di periodo archaico e classico. Diffusione, ideologia, committenza. Bari, Italy: Edipuglia; 2002. 244 p

[21] Krug A. Heilkunst und Heilkult: Medizin in der Antike. Munchen, Germany: Verlag H.C. Beck; 1993. 246 p

[22] Versakis F. Buildings in Asklepieion of Athens. Archaeologiki Ephimeris. 1913;**52**:52-74 (in Hellenic)

[23] Melfi M. Il santuario di Asclepio a Lebena. (Monografie della Scuola archeologica di Atene e delle missioni italiane in Oriente 19). Athens, Greece: Scuola archeologica italiana di Atene; 2007. 246 p

[24] Melfi M. I santuari di Asclepio in Grecia. I. In: Studia Archaeologica 157. Rome, Italy: L'Erma di Bretschneider; 2007. 578 p

[25] Gounaropoulou L, Hatzopoulos MB. Inscriptions of Makedonias I: Inscriptions Veroia (EKM). Athens 1998; In: Cormack JMR, editor. Unpublished Inscriptions from Beroea. Annual of the British School at Athens, Greece 39 (1938-1939); 1998. p. 96-97 (in Hellenic)

[26] Voutiras E. The cult of Asclepios in Ancient Macedonia. In: Ancient Macedonia V, Proceedings of the Conference of Ancient Macedonia; 10-15 October 1989; Thessaloniki, Greece: Volume 1; 1993. p. 251-265 (in Hellenic)

[27] Kavvadias P. The Sanctuary of Asclepius at Epidarus and the Treatment of the Patients. Athens, Greece: Perris Bros Press; 1900. 320 p. (in Hellenic)

[28] Jiuri-Levendopoulou E. The sanctuary of Zeus Ammon in Aphitis. In: Archaeologika Analekta Athinon III; 1971. pp. 356-367 (in Hellenic)

[29] Voutiras E. The cult of Asclepios in Ancient Macedonia. In: Ancient Macedonia V, Proceedings of the Conference of Ancient Macedonia; 10-14 October 1989; Thessaloniki, Greece; Foundation of the Peninsula of Haemus: Volume 1; 1993. pp. 251-265 (in Hellenic)

[30] Lilimpaki-Akamati M. Excavations in the channel area of Pella during 1988-1991. In: The Archaeological work of Macedonia and Thrace, Proceedings of the 5th Archaeological Symposium (1991), Thessaloniki, Greece; 1994. pp. 83-95 (in Hellenic)

[31] Pollak K. Die Heilkunde der Antike. Griechenland-Rom-Byzanz. Die Medizin in Bibel und Talmud. Wiesbaden, Germany: R Löwit; 1969. 383 p

[32] Moss G. Water and health: A forgotten connection? Perspectives in Public Health. 2010;**130**(5):227-232

[33] Dvorjetski E. Leisure, Pleasure and Healing Spa Culture and Medicine in Ancient Eastern Mediterranean. Leiden, Netherlands: Brill; 2007. 526 p

[34] Ginouvès R. 1962. Balaneutike: recherches sur le bain dans l'antiquite grecque. Paris; De Boccard; 2007. 512 p

[35] Papavramidou N, Papavramidis S, Christopoulou-Aletra H. Galen on obesity: Etiology, effects and treatment. World Journal of Surgery. 2004;**28**(6):631-635

[36] Thomas L. Scientific frontiers and national frontiers: A look ahead. Foreign Affairs. 1984;**62**(4):966-994

[37] Lypourlis D. Medicine in Ancient Greece. Thessaloniki, Greece: Epikentro; 2008. 290 p. (in Hellenic)

Chapter 5

Contamination of Emergency Medical Vehicles and Risk of Infection to Paramedic First Responders and Patients by Antibiotic-Resistant Bacteria: Risk Evaluation and Recommendations from Ambulance Case Studies

Andrew W. Taylor-Robinson

Abstract

Contamination of emergency medical vehicles with pathogenic microbes poses a potential threat to public health considering the many millions of ambulance responses that are made globally each year. This risk of infection is to the patients, to their companions who may travel with them, and to the paramedic first responders whose work involves pre- or inter-hospital transfer. This applies particularly to contamination by those infectious disease-causing microbes for which the threat is heightened because of their recognized resistance to leading antimicrobial agents. Determining the risks should facilitate the advancement of best practices to enhance infection control of routine outbreaks and during a major emergency such as a disease pandemic or a bioterrorism event. This may merit the introduction of amended guidelines for ambulance cleaning and disinfection to achieve more effective pre-hospital infection control among the worldwide community of emergency service providers.

Keywords: ambulance, antibiotic resistance, bacteria, best practice, contamination, emergency medical vehicle, first response, helicopter, infection control, MRSA, paramedic, pathogen, pre-hospital care, *Staphylococcus aureus*

1. Introduction

The emergency services work force, comprising paramedics, police, firefighters, and specialized rescue and response teams, carry out duties on a daily basis that are essential to individual safety and well-being and to the operational functioning of their local community. Beyond these regular, routine activities, emergency medical services also administer life-saving assistance following a critical incident. Against this background, of serious concern is amassing evidence from research case studies to suggest that emergency medical vehicles can act as carriers (so-called vectors) of pathogenic microorganisms, or microbes, thereby promoting human infectious disease transmission [1]. In order to reduce this identified risk, an extensive screening process for pathogens should be performed. Implementation of new or revised policies and procedures would help to safeguard against emergency services crew, equipment and vehicles being inadvertent infectious disease vectors, and so exacerbating the already profound health risks associated with pandemics, natural disasters and bioterrorism.

The contamination of emergency service vehicles with microbes from body fluids or excreta is shown by many recent international studies. This non-systematic review highlights the key findings of selected seminal reports. Raised levels of bacterial species potentially harmful to human health have been detected in a range of emergency medical vehicles and in distinct contexts [2–9]. Notably, ambulances were contaminated with the difficult-to-treat Gram-positive bacterium, methicillin-resistant *Staphylococcus aureus* (MRSA) [2, 3], which is resistant to the commonly used class of penicillin-related antibiotics. In 13 metropolitan ambulances test 49.9% of swab samples showed positive for bacteria; 0.9% were highly drug-resistant pathogenic strains: MRSA; methicillin-resistant coagulase-negative staphylococci (MRCoNS); and carbapenemase-producing *Klebsiella pneumoniae* (KPC) [4]. In a separate study on 21 ambulances, 47.6% of surface swabbings were positive for MRSA [5]. Further, "large numbers of microbes" were isolated from helicopter air ambulances [6], corroborated by more detailed findings from Australia [7]. Microbiological cultures swabbed from four ambulances demonstrated that "four of the seven species isolated were substantial nosocomial pathogens, and three of these four possess formidable antibiotic resistance patterns" [8]. Similarly, 49% of rural ambulances tested positive in at least one internal location for contamination with MRSA [9]. Gram-negative coliforms of a variety of genera including *Enterobacter*, *Klebsiella* and *Escherichia* were commonly detected [3], suggestive of contamination with fecal or soil matter.

Emergency care equipment was discovered to also be a source of contamination. Sphygmomanometer cuffs, stethoscopes and respirator masks in ambulances frequently carried enterococci and *S. aureus* [10]. In one study, 57% of patient-ready trauma equipment swabbed at six hospitals and three regional ambulance services in the UK tested positive for blood contamination [11]. Likewise, of 50 stethoscopes used by paramedics 32% tested positive for MRSA [12].

2. Examining emergency medical helicopters for bacterial contamination

The extent of the problem of bacterial contamination of ambulances is exemplified by a recent proof-of-concept case study that examined two helicopter air ambulances based in separate municipalities in Queensland, the north-eastern state of Australia [7]. Emergency medical helicopters were selected due to the dearth of research on this type of emergency service vehicle as a vector of infection transmission. The two aircraft made a collective 68 call responses over 3 months. These involved patient transfers for specialist care (66.2%), primary responses (23.4%) (including road traffic incidents, cardiac arrest and medical cases), neonatal transfer to or between maternity care facilities (8.8%), and one search and rescue case (1.5%). During the study period samples were collected by swabbing each helicopter on six occasions at approximately weekly intervals. The helicopter's flight log provided for every response details of travel distance, locations of departure, pick-up and destination, and number and role of persons in transit. The presence or absence of bacteria was correlated longitudinally against time with each of geographical location, intra-vehicle surfaces, flight schedules and cleaning timetables.

For each sampling, the helicopter's interior was swabbed in five sites considered by emergency response crew to have a high frequency of contact, either by

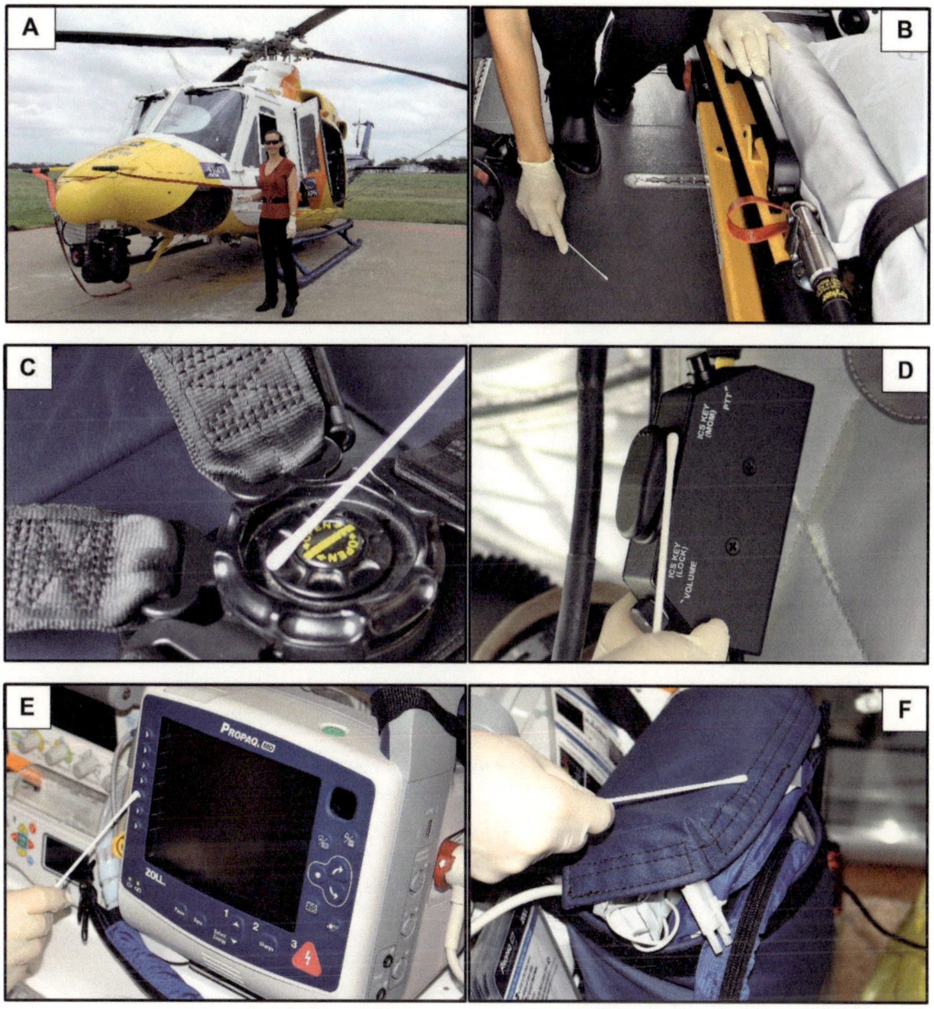

Figure 1.
Sites for microbiological swab sampling for detection of bacterial contamination inside a helicopter air ambulance. Following discussions with paramedic staff and pilots five areas of the aircraft (A) were considered to have a high frequency of contact by emergency crew and patients. These locations were: (B) the floor surface between the emergency crew seats and patient stretcher; (C) the seat belt buckle on the emergency crew seats; (D) the hand piece of the Citizens' Band radio; (E) the buttons on the display panel of the cardiac monitor/defibrillator; and (F) the blood pressure cuff storage bag [13].

themselves, patients and/or their companions, which thus present a raised risk of microbial contamination (**Figure 1**) [7, 13]. The diagnostic procedures followed were those approved by government regulatory bodies including the US Food and Drug Administration, comprising standard medical microbiology culture methods. These involved incubating the samples in a variety of selective media that differentiate positive bacterial colonies based on a difference in color. For example, after incubation on chromogenic MRSA agar for 24 hours at 35°C MRSA colonies are colored mauve whereas all other colonies appear blue, green or cream [14]. Confirmation of identity as either methicillin-resistant or multi-resistant bacteria was gained by conducting the disk diffusion (Kirby-Bauer) method on Mueller-Hinton agar [15]. This diagnostic screening was performed on all samples to determine the absence or presence of MRSA and multi-resistant *S. aureus*, vancomycin-resistant enterococci (VRE) and carbapenem-resistant enterobacteria (CRE), each of which is acknowledged to be a significant contributor to healthcare-associated infections [16, 17].

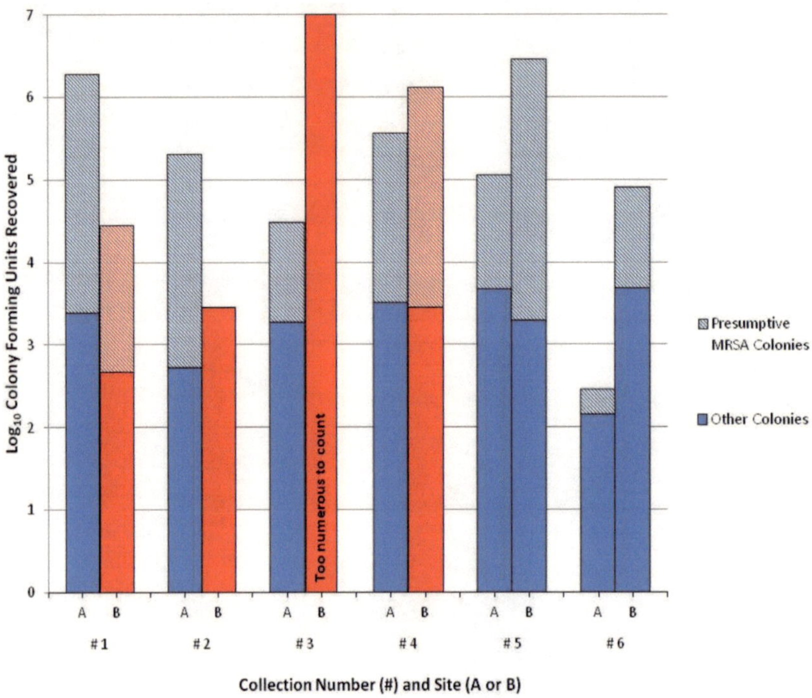

Figure 2.
Number and type of bacterial colonies recovered at each emergency service helicopter site for successive microbiological sampling periods. Bacterial counts are presented as Log_{10} of colony-forming units [7].

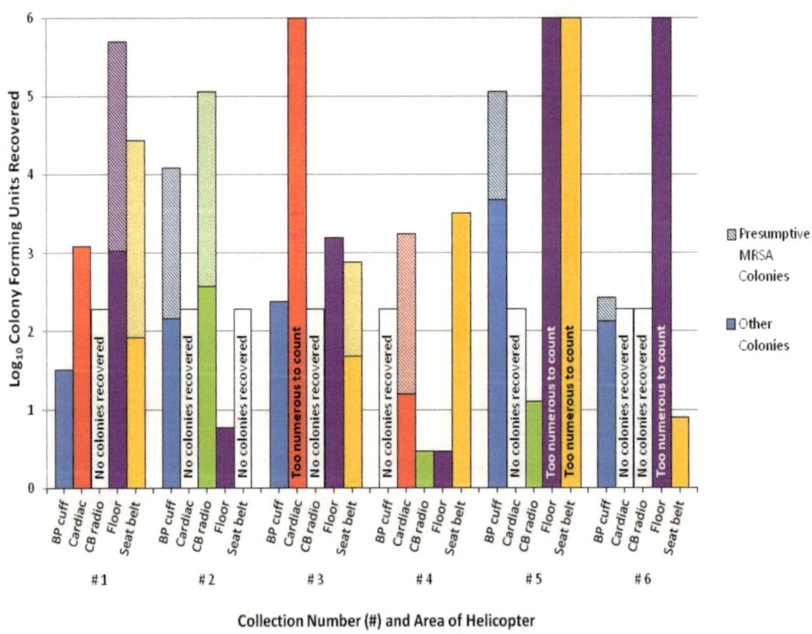

Figure 3.
Number and type of bacterial colonies recovered from different internal areas of the helicopter at emergency service site A for successive microbiological sampling periods. Bacterial counts are presented as Log_{10} of colony-forming units [7].

The equivalent antibiotic-susceptible organisms were also examined for as an indicator of the potential of the above antibiotic-resistant bacteria to be carried by these vehicles.

Both presumptive MRSA and other colonies were isolated from each helicopter at all but two sampling periods (**Figure 2**). Excluding occasions when selective media plates showed confluent bacterial growth the number of colony-forming units recovered from the two helicopters was similar (15,069 and 14,399). Of the presumptive colonies tested 18.7% were typed as *S. aureus*, 76.0% were determined to be other staphylococci (such as *S. haemolyticus* and *S. epidermidis*), and 5.3% were identified as other genera of bacteria [7]. Inside each helicopter, if separate swab sites were compared to each other or if the same swab site was examined over several sampling periods, various indicators of possible associations became apparent. For instance, typically the helicopter floor recorded a higher bacterial count, and the two-way radio and cardiac equipment comparatively lower counts, than for the other swabbed surfaces. Presumptive colonies were not recovered at all sampling periods, but they were isolated from all swab sites during the entirety of the study (**Figure 3**) [7].

As 94.7% of presumptive MRSA colonies tested were classified as *Staphylococcus* spp. the likelihood of MRSA existing inside emergency air ambulances is substantial. This is particularly so given that the prevalence of MRSA among emergency services crew is reported to exceed four times that of the general population [18]. The abundance of microbes recovered in this [7] and a prior study [6] suggests an increased risk of pathogen transfer between the vehicle, emergency services crew, patients and their companions. This serves to stress the need for standardized cleaning protocols as well as high quality staff training for their application.

3. Infection risks to paramedic first responders and patients

Previous research has detected MRSA in road-based ambulances in both metropolitan (47.6% of vehicle tests positive) [5] and rural areas (49% positive) [9]. An assortment of equipment used by emergency services crew has also shown frequent contamination [10–12]. Moreover, examination of nasal swabs demonstrated a disconcertingly raised prevalence of MRSA among paramedic first responders, 6.4%, much higher than the 1.5% MRSA colonization rate of the general public [18]. Of further concern, regarding a parallel issue of work-related stress it was reported that "paramedics ranked outbreaks of new and highly infectious disasters highest for fear and unfamiliarity" [19].

The existence of MRSA and multi-resistant *S. aureus* in emergency medical vehicles could pose a threat to the health of patients and their companions during and after the 4.4 and 32 million emergency ambulance responses each year in, respectively, Australia and the USA [20, 21], as well as to the paramedic first responders who work in these vehicles. This type and level of risk applies equally to emergency service crew in all nations worldwide. It would therefore appear that emergency medical helicopters may act as vectors of transmission of potentially deadly pathogens to the multiple thousands of patients that they transport between sites annually. By amplifying the frequency of response calls per vehicle type the implication is equally clear that road-based ambulances may spread infectious disease-causing microbes among the millions of patients that they transfer to and from hospitals each year. More broadly, inadequate infection control measures across all classes of emergency medical vehicle could exacerbate the major impact on public health of an infectious disease pandemic or bioterrorism event.

4. Cleaning and disinfection protocols for emergency medical vehicles

It is self-evident that surfaces or items that have come into contact with a patient's blood, body fluids, fecal matter or exposed skin should be considered as potentially contaminated. Since pathogenic microbes can survive outside the human body for extended periods the handling of contaminated objects is a means by which infection can spread [22]. A recurrent route of infection transmission is when a paramedic's gloved or ungloved hands touch a contaminated surface or medical equipment and/or there is patient contact with contaminated surfaces or items [23]. For this reason, it is imperative that items of patient care equipment (such as blood pressure cuffs, monitors, stethoscopes and stretchers) that make routine contact with skin and/or mucous membranes undergo a two-step cleaning and disinfection process following every response [24]. Defined as the simple removal of foreign and organic materials from a surface or object, cleaning using water, detergents and a scrubbing action physically removes but does not kill or prevent the growth of microbes. Conversely, disinfection kills or disables microbes present on contaminated surfaces, an operation that is customarily fulfilled with regulated chemical products [25].

The notable findings of one study showed that the number of sites contaminated inside an ambulance increased from 57% before cleaning and disinfection to 86% afterwards [3]. Hence, not only were many areas till contaminated with bacteria others that were previously uncontaminated became freshly contaminated as a result of poor cleaning technique acting as an inadvertent means of spread. The deficiency in performance of regular manual infection control protocols has been associated with operator error, principally concerning selection, formulation, distribution and contact time of the disinfectant [22, 23, 25]. Perspectives on improving effectiveness include staff training programs, continuing education, real-time feedback on the thoroughness of cleaning and disinfection procedures, routine microbiological inspection of surface hygiene, and the use of fluorescent markers or assays to ascertain the robustness of the process [25]. Although these actions can, separately and collectively, improve the efficacy of standard measures to decontaminate in the short-term, their sustainability is yet to be explored. The application of non-manual vehicle disinfection lowers the possibility of human errors linked to traditional cleaning methods and offers the prospect of more effective elimination of pathogens, thereby decreasing infection transmission [26]. However, at present definitive evidence is lacking to demonstrate the clinical effectiveness of non-touch or automated disinfection procedures, including those utilize steam cleaning, hydrogen peroxide or ultraviolet light irradiation, to eradicate or suppress infection rates in ambulances [27, 28].

5. Developing and implementing best practice guidelines for infection control

In view of the collective body of research which highlights that bacterial contamination of ambulances of all types is a frequent occurrence [2–12], the universal implementation of standardized, optimized infection control protocols is a high-priority public health provision [1]. Emergency services crew, their patients and companions have an elevated risk of contracting infection without there being in place clear guidelines and an understanding of, and adherence to, these protocols by paramedics [1, 24]. Compliance with best practices for cleaning and disinfecting inside emergency medical vehicles, equipment and supplies is an important consideration in aiming to prevent the spread of antibiotic-resistant bacteria in pre-hospital care settings. This may also drive the more general development of new or improved policies and procedures the adherence to which could decrease the day-to-day transmission of deadly pathogens and alleviate contagion by pandemic- or bioterrorism-related microbes.

In an attempt to reduce infectious disease transmission, reputedly antimicrobial fabrics have been used to manufacture uniforms for emergency medical service crew. However, in one short-term trial a suit made of one such novel fabric that was designed specifically to reduce contamination risks showed no significant difference in microbial contamination compared to garments made of standard materials [29].

Future investigations should aim to examine microbiological swab samples from a range of emergency service vehicles across a breadth of locations in order to detail and quantify the associated infection threat to the paramedic profession and to those to which they attend. This will help to define more clearly what strategies are needed to safeguard the provision of best practice and in case of natural disasters, pandemic outbreaks or possible bioterrorism events [30]. Integral to any mitigation recommendation should be professional development tailored to paramedic first responders in air ambulance helicopters and other emergency medical vehicles that is conducive to raising levels of awareness of infectious diseases and best practice training in infection control.

6. Discussion

Antibiotic-resistant bacteria are acknowledged to pose a profound and growing threat to human health, which, as recognized by the medical, nursing and paramedic professions, routinely cause a substantial proportion of healthcare-associated infections [31, 32]. Notwithstanding this realization, there is a knowledge gap in relation to the significance of antimicrobial resistance in pre-hospital emergency care [1], which is typically the primary point of patient contact.

While research from several countries has identified possible hazards [2–9], each of these preliminary studies focused on a single vehicle type. There is a shortfall in understanding of the relative contributions to potential infectious disease transmission of a wide spectrum of emergency service providers. The long-term objective should be to gauge the scale of contamination on or in emergency service vehicles, targeting police cars and fire trucks in addition to emergency medical vehicles. These include standard road-based ambulances, first response cars, motorcycle ambulances and helicopter air ambulances, as well as light aircraft used, for instance, by the Royal Flying Doctor Service in Australia to reach isolated patients in extremely remote locations. The data generated would be analyzed to assess the potential for uncontrolled disease spread, thereby facilitating the development of recommendations to minimize transmission risks for emergency response crews and for the communities that they serve.

Reflecting the bulk of findings to date, staphylococci form the focus of this chapter. However, the need to perform more research on Gram-negative coliforms as a source of potentially pathogenic bacterial contamination of emergency medical vehicles is highlighted.

7. Conclusion

The services of paramedics and other emergency medical professionals are a cornerstone of all civilized societies. Paradoxically, however, given the paramount importance of the role that this sector fulfills, there is a paucity of information on the risks of infectious disease transmission from contamination of vehicles, equipment or passengers by microbial pathogens. Assessment of potential threats to paramedics, patients and companions should be considered as an imperative in order to establish effective risk reduction interventions. Recent research has established that all types of emergency medical vehicle can act as vectors for infectious microbes. Items of equipment that are handled frequently by paramedics may be at heightened risk of contamination and should thus be prioritized for regular disinfection.

How to reduce the risk of antibiotic-resistant bacterial contamination of the interior of emergency medical vehicles is a pre-hospital care issue encountered on a daily basis but one which also has far-reaching implications in disaster management situations. Preventive measures intended to mitigate the threat of pathogenic bacterial transmission to ambulance staff, patients and their companions by ensuring a cleaner, safer medical environment exemplify paramedic industry best practice. Further detailed research is required to determine the potential risk of infection transmission among different vehicle fleets and under varied conditions of use. This may underpin the establishment and implementation of new or revised policies and protocols for cleaning and disinfection schedules. Committing to such action should fortify the paramedic sector's mission to save lives, speed recovery and serve the community through providing the highest standards of rapid response critical care.

Acknowledgements

The author's research referred to herein received financial support from Central Queensland University's Research Development and Incentives Program; Merit Grant number 0980022829, 'Antibiotic-resistant bacterial contamination of emergency medical vehicles — is there a risk to patients and providers?'. The participation of the emergency helicopter service providers RACQ Capricorn Rescue and CareFlight is gratefully acknowledged. Present and former colleagues Sandrine Maguire, Brian Maguire and Anthony Weber are warmly thanked for sharing their expert views over many years.

Conflicts of interest

The author declares no competing issues of interest.

Author details

Andrew W. Taylor-Robinson
Infectious Diseases Research Group, School of Health, Medical and Applied Sciences, Central Queensland University, Brisbane, QLD, Australia

Address all correspondence to: a.taylor-robinson@cqu.edu.au

IntechOpen

© 2019 The Author(s). Licensee IntechOpen. This chapter is distributed under the terms of the Creative Commons Attribution License (http://creativecommons.org/licenses/by/3.0), which permits unrestricted use, distribution, and reproduction in any medium, provided the original work is properly cited.

References

[1] Makiela S, Weber A, Maguire BJ, Taylor-Robinson AW. Infection control protocols: Is it time to clean up our act? The Australasian Journal of Paramedicine. 2018;**15**(3):5-8

[2] Eibicht S, Vogel U. Meticillin-resistant *Staphylococcus aureus* (MRSA) contamination of ambulance cars after short term transport of MRSA-colonised patients is restricted to the stretcher. The Journal of Hospital Infection. 2011;**78**(3):221-225

[3] Nigam Y, Cutter J. A preliminary investigation into bacterial contamination of Welsh emergency ambulances. Emergency Medicine Journal. 2003;**20**(5):479-482

[4] Noh H, Shin SD, Kim NJ, Ro YS, Oh HS, et al. Risk stratification-based surveillance of bacterial contamination in metropolitan ambulances. Journal of Korean Medical Science. 2011;**26**(1):124-130

[5] Roline CE, Crumpecker C, Dunn TM. Can methicillin-resistant *Staphylococcus aureus* be found in an ambulance fleet? Prehospital Emergency Care. 2007;**11**(2):241-244

[6] Galtelli M, Deschamp C, Rogers J. An assessment of the prevalence of pathogenic microorganisms in the rotor wing air ambulance: One program's findings. Air Medical Journal. 2006;**25**(2):81-84

[7] Makiela S, Taylor-Robinson AW, Weber A, Maguire BJ. A preliminary assessment of contamination of emergency service helicopters with MRSA and multi-resistant *Staphylococcus aureus*. Emergency Medicine: Open Access. 2016;**6**(1):304-310

[8] Alves DW, Bissell RA. Bacterial pathogens in ambulances: Results of unannounced sample collection. Prehospital Emergency Care. 2008;**12**(2):218-224

[9] Brown R, Minnon J, Schneider S, Vaughn J. Prevalence of methicillin-resistant *Staphylococcus aureus* in ambulances in southern Maine. Prehospital Emergency Care. 2010;**14**(2):176-181

[10] Kober P, Labes H, Möller H, Hülsse C, Kramer A. Hygiene status of ambulances and equipment in rescue services. Anästhesiologie, Intensivmedizin, Notfallmedizin, Schmerztherapie: AINS. 2001;**36**(1): 25-30. (Article in German)

[11] Lee J, Levy M, Walker A. Use of a forensic technique to identify blood contamination of emergency department and ambulance trauma equipment. Emergency Medicine Journal. 2006;**23**(1):73-75

[12] Merlin MA, Wong ML, Pryor PW, Rynn K, Marques-Baptista A, et al. Prevalence of methicillin-resistant *Staphylococcus aureus* on the stethoscopes of emergency medical services providers. Prehospital Emergency Care. 2009;**13**(1):71-74

[13] Taylor-Robinson AW, Makiela S. Determining the risk of antibiotic-resistant bacterial contamination of emergency medical vehicles and paramedic personnel: Conclusions from a helicopter air ambulance case study. Journal of Community Medicine. 2019;**2**(1):1-5

[14] Stoakes L, Reyes R, Daniel J, Lennox G, John MA, et al. Prospective comparison of a new chromogenic medium, MRSA *Select*, to CHROMagar MRSA and mannitol-salt medium supplemented with oxacillin or cefoxitin for detection of methicillin-resistant *Staphylococcus aureus*. Journal of Clinical Microbiology. 2006;**44**(2):637-639

[15] Skov R, Smyth R, Larsen AR, Bolmstrom A, Karlsson A, et al. Phenotypic detection of methicillin resistance in *Staphylococcus aureus* by disk diffusion testing and Etest on Mueller-Hinton agar. Journal of Clinical Microbiology. 2006;**44**(12):4395-4399

[16] Fernando SA, Gray TJ, Gottlieb T. Healthcare-acquired infections: Prevention strategies. Internal Medicine Journal. 2017;**47**(12):1341-1351

[17] Goyal S, Khot SC, Ramachandran V, Shah KP, Musher DM. Bacterial contamination of medical providers' white coats and surgical scrubs: A systematic review. American Journal of Infection Control. 2019; pii: S0196-6553(19)30053-7. DOI: 10.1016/j.ajic.2019.01.012. [Epub ahead of print]

[18] Amiry AA, Bissell RA, Maguire BJ, Alves DW. Methicillin-resistant *Staphylococcus aureus* nasal colonization prevalence among emergency medical services personnel. Prehospital and Disaster Medicine. 2013;**28**(4):1-5

[19] Smith EC, Burkle FM, Archer FL. Fear, familiarity, and the perception of risk: A quantitative analysis of disaster-specific concerns of paramedics. Disaster Medicine and Public Health Preparedness. 2011;**5**(1):46-53

[20] Australian Government Productivity Commission. Report on Government Services. 2018. Available from: https://www.pc.gov.au/research/ongoing/report-on-government-services/2018/health/ambulance-services/rogs-2018-parte-chapter11.pdf [Accessed: 24 May 2019]

[21] Maguire BJ, Walz BJ. Current emergency medical services workforce issues in the United States. Journal of Emergency Management. 2004;**2**(1):17-26

[22] Siegel JD, Rhinehart E, Jackson M, Chiarello L, and the Healthcare Infection Control Practices Advisory Committee. Guideline for Isolation Precautions: Preventing Transmission of Infectious Agents in Healthcare Settings. 2007. Available from: http://www.cdc.gov/ncidod/dhqp/pdf/isolation2007.pdf [Accessed: 24 May 2019]

[23] Muto CA, Jernigan JA, Ostrowsky BE, Richet HM, Jarvis WR, et al. SHEA guideline for preventing nosocomial transmission of multidrug-resistant strains of *Staphylococcus aureus* and *Enterococcus*. Infection Control and Hospital Epidemiology. 2003;**24**(5):362-386

[24] Fleming J. EMS equipment and transport vehicle cleaning and disinfection: Challenges and best practices. EMS World. 2009. Available from: https://www.emsworld.com/article/10320653/ems-equipment-and-transport-vehicle-cleaning-and-disinfection-challenges-best-practices [Accessed: 24 May 2019]

[25] Public Health Ontario, Provincial Infectious Diseases Advisory Committee. Best Practices for Environmental Cleaning for Prevention and Control of Infections in All Health Care Settings. 3rd ed. Toronto: Queen's Printer for Ontario; 2018

[26] Cimon K, Argáez C. Non-Manual Disinfection Techniques for Ambulances: Clinical Effectiveness and Guidelines. Ottawa: Canadian Agency for Drugs and Technologies in Health; 2018. Available from: https://www.cadth.ca/sites/default/files/pdf/htis/2018/RB1197%20Non-Manual%20Disinfection%20Final.pdf [Accessed: 24 May 2019]

[27] Marra AR, Schweizer ML, Edmond MB. No-touch disinfection methods to decrease multidrug-resistant organism infections: A systematic review and meta-analysis. Infection Control and Hospital Epidemiology. 2018;**39**(1):20-31

[28] Lindsley WG, McClelland TL, Neu DT, Martin SB Jr. Mead KR, et al. Ambulance disinfection using ultraviolet germicidal irradiation (UVGI): Effects of fixture location and surface reflectivity. Journal of Occupational and Environmental Hygiene. 2018;**15**(1):1-12

[29] Groß R, Hübner N, Assadian O, Jibson B, Kramer A. Pilot study on the microbial contamination of conventional vs. silver-impregnated uniforms worn by ambulance personnel during one week of emergency medical service. GMS Krankenhaushygiene Interdisziplinär. 2010;**5**(2):Doc09

[30] Maguire BJ, Dean S, Bissell RA, Walz BJ, Bumbak AK. Epidemic and bioterrorism preparation among emergency medical services systems. Prehospital and Disaster Medicine. 2007;**22**(3):237-242

[31] Ferri M, Ranucci E, Romagnoli P, Giaccone V. Antimicrobial resistance: A global emerging threat to public health systems. Critical Reviews in Food Science and Nutrition. 2017;**57**(13):2857-2876

[32] Centers for Disease Control and Prevention. About Antimicrobial Resistance. 2018. Available from: http://cdc.gov/drugresistance/about.html [Accessed: 24 May 2019]

Section 3

Infection Control Strategies

Chapter 6

Medical Management of Chronic Plaque Psoriasis in the Modern Age

Teodora-Larisa Timis, Daniela-Rodica Mitrea and Ioan-Alexandru Florian

Abstract

Despite its frequency, psoriasis is still a difficult pathology to manage, in no small part due to the wide number of therapeutic choices available. These range from topical medicine to systemic drugs to more targeted agents such as biological therapies. All medical personnel involved in the treatment of psoriasis patients should be aware of these methods and apply them accordingly. Even though all patients may benefit from specific treatment options, these differ in regard to posology, monitoring, interactions and contraindications. Moreover, due to the adverse effects and drug interactions of some of these agents, not all patients are suitable candidates for each of therapies discussed. Therefore, nurses, trainees, general practitioners and dermatologists must carefully select the most appropriate therapy based on the characteristics of each patient, severity of the pathology, comorbidities and coexistent medications. This review aims to offer an updated, pragmatic insight into the modern management of patients with moderate-to-severe psoriasis.

Keywords: psoriasis, T cells, immunomodulators, keratinocytes, phototherapy, systemic therapies, biologic agents

1. Introduction and short history

Psoriasis is defined as chronic inflammatory systemic ailment, affecting the teguments foremost, and characterized by important genetic and immune constituents. The most common form is represented by psoriasis vulgaris, affecting every race and all ages, most often between the ages of 50 and 69 years, concerning at least 100 million individuals worldwide [1, 2]. It is a potentially devastating disorder with a progressive natural course, associated with multiple comorbidities and typified by underlying immunologic and inflammatory elements [3]. Despite it being a convoluted pathology with an incompletely elucidated pathogenesis, it has been shown that the environment, immune system and genetic predisposition all play a decisive role in triggering the psoriasis cascade [4]. As of today, treating psoriasis remains a demanding endeavour, merely attending the symptoms and ignoring the principal cause. Medical management is satiated by a wide variety of choices with fluctuating efficiency, for example, topical therapies, phototherapy, systemic drugs and biological agents [5]. It is fathomable that choosing the most appropriate treatment scheme for each individual can oftentimes be perplexing or even disheartening. Nevertheless, the treatment involved should imply a multidisciplinary course

IntechOpen

of action, with psychologists, rheumatologists and dermatologists collaborating in order to deliver the best possible care, with the most satisfactory outcome.

To properly understand the breakthroughs of modern treatment of psoriasis, it might be worthwhile to glance over the history of this complicated disease. The first reported cases were identified in ancient Greece, many of the description written by Hippocrates (460–377 BC) himself [6, 7]. Portrayals of psoriasis can also be traced back to the times of the Old Testament, wherein people suffering from such skin disorders were publicly ostracized since they were considered punished by divinity. Numerous historians acknowledge Celsus (ca. 25 BC–45 AD) as documenting the first clinical description of papulosquamous diseases, whereas Galen (133–200 AD) first utilized the term psoriasis [6, 8, 9]. However, his depiction was inconsistent regarding the disorder that we now know as psoriasis. He described it as a pruritic, scaly skin illness of the eyelids and scrotum, probably referred to as today as seborrheic dermatitis. Nevertheless, the unselective grouping together of all inflammatory skin disorders contributed to the stigmatization of psoriasis patients. During the Middle Ages, when it was believed that psoriasis was as contagious as leprosy, these patients were mandated to carry a chime or clapper that would announce their approach. Furthermore, they had to wear a special garment and could only eat or come into physical contact with others considered lepers.

In the dawn of the nineteenth century, Willan expanded on Celsus's explanations of papulosquamous afflictions by describing characteristics we know considered compatible with psoriasis. Even so, he labelled modern psoriasis as 'lepra vulgaris', which maintained the confusion between these two distinct diseases [6, 7, 10]. Afterwards, there was an incongruity when referring to these pathologies, as authors could not properly agree on which term to use. Ultimately, Gibert corroborated Willan's description with the term psoriasis, putting an end to some of the perplexity and guiding to an improved awareness and understanding of psoriatic patients. Heinrich Auspitz (1835–1886) noticed the papillary bleeding that appeared after removing the scale of psoriatic lesions, currently referred to as the Auspitz sign (or bloody dew phenomenon) [6, 7, 11, 12]. In 1877, Heinrich Köbner (1838–1904) defined the sign that carries his name, specifically the occurrence of a psoriatic lesion within the location of a physical injury. After two more decades, in 1898, William Munro (1863–1908) described the microabscesses that appear in psoriasis, otherwise known as Munro's abscesses. The beginning of the twentieth century led to further advancements in the understanding of psoriatic lesions. In 1910, Leo von Zumbusch (1874–1940) was the first to note generalized pustular psoriasis, now called the von Zumbusch disease [6, 13]. Among other descriptions was also the one of the Russian dermatologist D.L. Woronoff in 1926 regarding a pale halo now known as the 'Woronoff ring' enclosing a plaque of psoriasis [7, 14]. The characterization of the Auspitz sign, Köbner's phenomenon, Munro's abscess, and pustular psoriasis, as well as the Woronoff ring made it possible for practitioners to more easily identify patients with psoriasis.

The next discoveries furthered our understanding of pathophysiology, especially concerning epidermal hyperplasia and keratinocytes' cell cycle shortening by van Scott and Ekel in 1963, followed by the role of the immune system by Gubner in 1951 and Muller in 1979 [6, 7]. However, there is still much to be learned about this complex disease and its intricate mechanisms.

The treatment of psoriasis also varied across the ages, from arsenic and ammoniated mercury in the nineteenth century (which both had a comparable toxic potential), to chrysarobin, anthralin and coal tars in the late nineteenth and early twentieth centuries, reaching to corticosteroids, methotrexate and PUVA in the middle of the last century [6, 7, 10, 15]. In what follows, we describe the modern forms of therapy which have been scientifically proven to ameliorate the symptoms in psoriasis.

2. Management of psoriasis

In the past few years, countless achievements have been made in grasping the intricate physiopathological contrivances of psoriasis. Studies repeatedly demonstrated that it is a chronic, systemic immune-mediated ailment, the dermatologic manifestation representing its most debilitating aspect, usually followed by joint involvement. However, the explicit mechanisms of this process have not been untangled. Even so, it appears that the myeloid dendritic cells begin producing interleukins such as IL-12, IL-23 and TNF-α prior to a minor traumatic injury that perform as chemoattractants for the T helper Th-1 and Th-17 cells [16, 17]. In the next step, these cells will raise the production of psoriatic cytokines such as IL-17 within the site of injury, hence increasing the keratinocytes' turnover and eventually piloting towards the cutaneous symptoms of psoriasis [18–21]. Also, the proinflammatory substances may extend into the bloodstream with a significant influence on insulin signalling, angiogenesis, lipogenesis or adipogenesis, which will ultimately lead to comorbidities such as obesity and dyslipidaemia, hypertension, depression and type 2 diabetes mellitus [3, 22]. Grasping the mechanisms of psoriasis is the utmost step in offering the best available therapy.

Topical therapy as the only form of treatment has demonstrated a mediocre rate of improvement, with patients often describing ongoing clinical symptoms, for instance, redness, pruritus or scales [23]. One survey targeted to such patients showed that 40% of cases with a mild disease, circa 50% of those with moderate psoriasis and well above 40% with the severe form were discontented with the recommended topical therapies. The lowermost treatment satisfaction quotients were found in the topical medications versus systemic and phototherapy group [24]. Should topical therapy in itself fail to achieve the expected outcome, practitioners have to be ready for alternative strategies, such as systemic and biological therapies.

2.1 Topical therapy

Topical therapies are recommended in mild psoriasis, when the affected body surface area is below 10% [25].

2.1.1 Anthralin

Anthralin via mitochondrial dysfunction might reduce the proliferation of keratinocytes and re-establish cell differentiation. As such, it is used to treat the localized plaques that are covered with thick scales localized either on body or the scalp that have failed to clear with other treatments. It is applied on the affected areas in concentration of 1%, and it is left between 20 min and 1 h before removal [26].

Among the adverse effects, the common is skin irritation or staining of the adjoining skin [25].

2.1.2 Coal tar

Coal tar seems to reduce hyperproliferation of keratinocytes by supressing DNA synthesis, and it has exhibited efficacy on chronic plaque psoriasis, palmoplantar psoriasis or scalp psoriasis, improving the general aspect of the psoriasis plaque after 1 month of treatment. It appears as though the remission period of the lesions persists longer than that with other topical treatments [25].

Adverse effects number odour, staining, contact dermatitis, erythema and folliculitis.

It can be used during pregnancy, but in children caution is advertised [27].

2.1.3 Salicylic acid

Salicylic acid triggers desquamation of corneocytes via lowering intracellular cohesion between the cells of the stratum corneum. It can be applied in creams, ointments or lotions in concentrations between 2 and 6%.

The most notable adverse effect mentioned while using salicylic acid is the potential systemic intoxication [28].

It is safe to utilize during pregnancy, but in children, because of the systemic absorption, it should be avoided [25].

2.1.4 Calcineurin

Calcineurin inhibitors like tacrolimus, pimecrolimus and sirolimus supress the production of the inflammatory substances that seem accountable for the skin lesions in psoriasis. It is found in concentration of 0.3% gel or 0.5% cream [29].

As side effects, the most common is stinging sensation or contact dermatitis.

It can be used in children older than 2 years old [25].

2.1.5 Topical retinoids tazarotene and bexarotene

Topical retinoids tazarotene and bexarotene downregulate the turnover by altering transcription of genes in keratinocytes upon transportation within the nucleus, after binding to retinoic acid on the cell membrane. Furthermore, it reduces the hyperproliferation of keratinocytes; it regulates the differentiation and reduces inflammation [30].

It can be applied as a cream in concentration of 0.1 and 0.05%, and when used on the nails, it seems to improve the onycholysis, pitting and salmon patches [25].

It is contraindicated during pregnancy, but it is permitted to be used in children [31].

2.1.6 Topical corticosteroids

Topical corticosteroids display immunosuppressive, anti-inflammatory, anti-proliferative and vasoactive action. They are categorized based on their potency, from low-potency to very potent corticosteroids. When considering the potency and the vehicle, disease severity, patient preference and sites of lesions must be taken into account [25]. They can be found as creams, ointments, gel, solutions, nail lacquer, foams or shampoos applied on the skin, scalp or nails.

Skin atrophy, telangiectasia as well as secondary infection are the most notable side effects.

Corticosteroids can be used during pregnancy but are not recommended in children under 2 years old [32].

2.1.7 Vitamin D

Vitamin D analogues calcitriol, tacalcitol, maxacalcitol, paricalcitol and becocalcidiol decrease keratinocyte proliferation, inflammation or keratinization [33]. They can be applied on the skin, scalp or nails and are found as creams, ointments or scalp lotions.

The most common side effect is skin irritation. Very rare hypercalcemia, hypercalciuria and parathyroid hormone suppression have been described.

Vitamin D analogues are contraindicated in patients with hypercalcemia or in pregnancy, but they can be used in children while not exceeding the dose of 50 g/week [34].

2.2 Phototherapy in psoriasis

Ultraviolets either from the sun or artificial light play a significant role in treating psoriasis mainly by supressing activated T cells, independently on the cell subpopulation involved in the disease [25]. It has been shown that NB-UVB is the most utilized phototherapeutical approach, inducing clinical and histopathological resolution of moderate-to-severe plaque psoriasis by exerting a cytotoxic effect on epidermal T cells [35, 36]. This apoptotic effect on T cells depends mostly on the penetration of the NB-UVB within the lesion, penetration that on the one hand depends on the wavelength and on the other the depth of the skin lesion [37]. Understanding that the T cells responsible for psoriasis are situated along the dermal-epidermal junction and within the epidermis, it has been determined that the optimal wavelength spectrum should range between 290 and 313 nm [38]. Currently, NB-UVB is the most common approached used worldwide, and it can be regarded as the gold standard in therapy for treating moderate-to-severe plaque psoriasis [39].

2.3 Systemic therapies

2.3.1 Methotrexate

Methotrexate is a folic acid analogue employed in psoriasis for its anti-proliferative, anti-inflammatory and immunosuppressive actions [40].

Dosage and administration. Methotrexate comes as a self-injectable solution administered by the patient weekly, with the added proposal of coupling with folic acid supplements. Initiation dosage is typically 10–25 mg once per week. Maximum dose should not surpass 30 mg/week. Folate intake should be about 1–5 mg daily, except on the day of methotrexate intake [41].

Adverse effects. In case of pregnancy, it may lead to foetal death or to teratogenic effects; also, it can be toxic to the gastrointestinal tube, liver and kidneys, and it can cause myelosuppression, malignant lymphomas, pulmonary fibrosis, severe infections, fatigue, headaches, alopecia or oligospermia [42, 43].

Laboratory tests recommended. To start therapy with methotrexate correspondingly, the following evaluations are compulsory: physical exam, patient history, QuantiFERON-TB Gold for latent TB infection, complete blood count with differential and thrombocytes count, renal function tests, hepatic enzymes and pregnancy test.

Drug interactions. Methotrexate has been shown to interact with cyclosporine, proton pump inhibitors, oral antibiotics, salicylates, mercaptopurine, nonsteroidal anti-inflammatory drugs, cisplatin, probenecid, phenylbutazone, sulfonamides, theophylline, live vaccines, retinoids and azathioprine [43].

As anticipated, this drug is contraindicated in pregnancy and while breastfeeding due to its teratogenic effects. Therefore, the use of contraception is highly advocated in the course of treatment. Other contraindications include blood dyscrasia, chronic liver disease, immune deficiency syndromes or alcohol abuse [44].

2.3.2 Cyclosporine

Cyclosporine is a calcineurin inhibitor agent that is used in psoriasis for its immunosuppressing action and its capability to prevent the T cell proliferation by reversibly inhibiting the activation of CD4+ T cells, leading to a block on the synthesis of interleukin 2 [45].

Dosage and administration. To induct psoriasis remission, the everyday dosage varies between 2.5 and 5 mg/kg, administered in two divided doses each day. Experts recommend it not be used continuously for longer than 1 whole year [46].

Adverse effects. Among the most important reported adverse effects of cyclosporine are renal toxicity, structural kidney damage, hypertension, liver toxicity, severe infections, high potassium levels, low magnesium levels, acne, tremors, headache, pneumonitis and gastrointestinal toxicity [47, 48].

Laboratory tests recommended. Physical exam, patient history, QuantiFERON-TB Gold for latent TB infection, renal function tests, complete blood count with differential and platelet count, magnesium level, potassium level, uric acid, lipids, glycaemia, bilirubin and liver enzymes are necessary before initiating therapy. The serum creatinine should be measured on two distinct occasions. Contraception has to be ensured.

Drug interactions. Cyclosporine interacts with a large number of drugs such as antibiotics (ciprofloxacin, gentamicin, tobramycin, vancomycin, trimethoprim with sulfamethoxazole, azithromycin, erythromycin), nonsteroidal anti-inflammatory drugs, antifungals (amphotericin B, ketoconazole, fluconazole, itraconazole, terbinafine), ranitidine, cimetidine, birth control pills, tacrolimus, methotrexate, methylprednisone, allopurinol, colchicine, fenofibrate, gemfibrozil, statins, calcium channel blockers, amiodarone, bromocriptine, anticonvulsants (carbamazepine, oxcarbazepine, phenobarbital), protease inhibitors (indinavir, nelfinavir, ritonavir, saquinavir) and octreotide [48].

It is contraindicated in the case of poorly controlled arterial hypertension, known malignancies or renal dysfunctions. As of yet, there have not been enough studies performed in humans to certify whether the drug affects the foetus or not. Nonetheless, the treatment is still to be avoided in pregnant women due to the role calcineurin inhibitors are believed to play in neural development. As such, cyclosporine should only be used in pregnancy if the benefits justify the hypothetical risk to the foetus [49].

2.3.3 Acitretin

Acitretin is a retinoid agent with substantial immunomodulatory and anti-inflammatory effects, advocated in psoriasis for its capacity to modulate the proliferation and differentiation of keratinocytes [50].

Dosage and administration. Acitretin is taken in a single oral dose, alongside the main meal. Therapeutic dosage varies between 25 and 50 mg/day. A simultaneous topical therapy is also suggested due to the slow onset of action, needing as long as 3–6 months for a maximal response to acitretin [51].

Adverse effects. It can cause serious teratogenic effects on the exposed foetus, mucocutaneous dryness, hypertriglyceridemia, hepatotoxicity, toxic hepatitis, pancreatitis, hyperostosis, intracranial hypertension, alopecia, arthralgia and fatigue [52].

Laboratory tests recommended. It is compulsory to take a pregnancy test before initiating the treatment; liver enzymes, lipid profile, renal function and complete blood count should also be included.

Drug interactions. Acitretin interacts with retinoic acid supplements, methotrexate, doxycycline, oral retinoids and phenytoin [53].

The high teratogenicity of retinoids severely restricts their use in fertile women who should be appropriately counselled on the methods and importance of contraception [54]. Moreover, pregnancy should be circumvented for at least 3 years after halting treatment. A pregnancy test is to be performed regularly every 3 months during the course of therapy.

2.3.4 Fumaric acid esters and dimethyl fumarate

Fumaric acid esters and dimethyl fumarate have been employed in the treatment of psoriasis for five decades, with substantial outcomes for patients [55]. Seemingly, dimethyl fumarate affects multiple cytokines and lymphocyte pathways, i.e. inhibiting the nuclear translocation and the transcriptional activity of the nuclear factor kappa-light-chain-enhancer of activated B-cells through its interaction with the intracellular reduced glutathione. It also transforms the T helper cells from the Th1 and the Th17 profile to a Th2 phenotype, subsequently reducing cytokine production and the proliferation of epithelial cells [56].

Dosage and administration. It is available as gastro-resistant tablets, being recommended to start with a low initial dose that may be subsequently increased in the following manner: in the first week, it is advised to take one 30 mg tablet, in the second week one 30 mg tablet can be taken twice daily, and during the third week one 30 mg tablet is taken three times per day. From the fourth week onwards, it can be switched to one 120 mg tablet, taken in the evening. Depending on the results, this dose can be increased with one 120 mg tablet per week, but the maximum daily dose should not exceed 720 mg [57].

Adverse effects. Among more regularly reported events are gastrointestinal disorders, flushing, haematological disturbances (lymphopenia, leukopenia, eosinophilia), loss of appetite, headache, paraesthesia, proteinuria, renal failure, Fanconi syndrome and fatigue [58].

Reference tests. Complete blood count, renal function and liver enzymes should be included.

Drug interactions. Fumaric acid esters may interact with live vaccines, methotrexate, retinoids, cyclosporine, aminoglycosides, lithium, diuretics and nonsteroidal anti-inflammatory drugs [59].

2.3.5 Apremilast

Apremilast, operating as a selective inhibitor of phosphodiesterase 4, on the one hand downregulates the expression of specific proinflammatory cytokines like IL-17, IL-23 and TNF-α that each plays a crucial role in the pathophysiological chain of events in psoriasis. On the other hand, using the same mechanism, it increases the expression of anti-inflammatory cytokines such as IL-10 [59].

Dosage and administration. Presented in tablet form, apremilast is administered orally, with an indicated dose of 30 mg two times per day. The treatment should begin with a low starting dose of 10 mg in the morning, and then from the second day of therapy onward the dosage is increased daily by 10 mg until reaching the therapeutic dose of 30 mg twice daily [60, 61].

Adverse effects. Diarrhoea, nausea and vomiting, depression and weight loss are the most frequently noted adverse effects of apremilast [62].

Laboratory tests recommended. Physical exam, patient history (with an emphasis on psychiatric disorders such as depression), renal function and liver enzymes should be performed.

Drug interactions. Apremilast interacts with cytochrome P450 enzyme inducers such as rifampin, phenobarbital, carbamazepine and phenytoin [61].

Patients over 65 years old appear to be more vulnerable to develop the aforementioned side effects. Hence, supervision is very important in these cases, patients being warned regarding undesirable events. They should also be instructed not to reduce or suspend the medication by themselves, but to address their treating physician [62].

2.4 Biologic therapies

2.4.1 The anti-TNF-α agents

The anti-TNF-α agents etanercept, adalimumab, infliximab and certolizumab have been developed to expressly inhibit the TNF-α signalling pathway, thereby lessening its inflammatory properties. Etanercept is a recombinant TNF-α receptor that impedes TNF-α function by operating as a decoy receptor that attaches to TNF. Adalimumab is an entirely humanized antibody of TNF-α, where infliximab is a mouse-human chimeric antibody. Certolizumab represents a distinctive anti-TNF-α antibody that does not include the Fc portion [63, 64].

Dosage and administration. Etanercept, adalimumab and certolizumab are given via subcutaneous injection either weekly or once every two weeks. Infliximab is administered via intravenous infusion every 8 weeks. **Table 1** presents the dosage and the administration method for the abovementioned anti-TNF-α agents [65–68].

Adverse effects. Among the serious side effects encountered while using any of the mentioned anti-TNF-α agents are severe infections, lymphomas or other malignancies and even the reactivation of the tuberculosis or hepatitis B virus. While using etanercept, adalimumab or certolizumab, the most usual local reactions are pain, swelling, haemorrhage or erythema at the place of injection; however, the intensity of these symptoms will diminish with continued treatment. Patients should be advised not to accept taking live vaccinations for the duration of the therapy. There have been reported cases of CNS demyelinating pathologies (e.g. multiple sclerosis, optic neuritis) or peripheral nerve demyelinating disease (Guillain-Barré syndrome). Patients are advised to suspend the therapy in these cases [3, 65–68].

Laboratory tests recommended. Physical exam and history, complete blood count, liver function, renal function, viral hepatitis screening and tuberculosis testing should be performed prior to anti-TNF-α treatment initiation.

Drug interactions. Other biologic therapies, live vaccines, anakinra and abatacept, were noticed to interact with anti-TNF-α drugs [65–68].

Certolizumab has been approved by the FDA for pregnant women. Data collected thus far has validated neither additional teratogenic effects when compared to the general population, nor a greater risk of foetal death [69].

2.4.2 The anti-IL-12/23 agents

The anti-IL-12/23 agents comprise ustekinumab, guselkumab and tildrakizumab. Il-23 is a heterodimeric cytokine incorporating two subunits: the p19 subunit, which is connected to the p40 subunit, the latest being shared with IL-12. Il-23 is the main actor prompting the activation of the T helper 17 inflammatory pathway, whereas IL-12 plays the chief role in Th-1 differentiation and proliferation. Ustekinumab is a biologic agent aiming for the p40 common domain of IL-12 and IL-23, hence preventing their interaction with their receptor. Contrariwise, guselkumab and tildrakizumab target the p19 subunit of IL-23, thus obstructing the signalling pathway associated with the immunopathogenesis of psoriasis [70–72].

Dosage and administration. Ustekinumab, guselkumab and tildrakizumab are delivered as prefilled syringes with subcutaneous administration. The induction phase lasts 1 month, being then ensued by the maintenance phase. In this phase, an injection is administered once every 8 or 12 weeks. **Table 2** presents the respective posology for the aforementioned biologic agents [73–75].

Biologic agent	Posology
Etanercept	50 mg × 1 twice a week during the induction phase (the first 3 months), thereafter only one injection weekly
Adalimumab	40 mg × 2 at week 0, afterwards 40 mg × 1 administered every 14 days
Infliximab	5 mg/kg is administered via intravenous infusion at weeks 0, 2 and 6 and after that every 8 weeks
Certolizumab	200 mg × 2 administered subcutaneously at weeks 2 and 4, followed by a 200 mg × 1 dose weekly

Table 1.
Anti-TNF-α agents. Posology.

Biologic agent	Posology
Ustekinumab	45 mg × 1 administered at weeks 0 and 4 and at every 12 weeks subsequently
Guselkumab	100 mg × 1 administered at weeks 0 and 4 and at every 8 weeks afterwards
Tildrakizumab	100 mg × 1 administered at week 0 and 4 and every 12 weeks thereafter

Table 2.
Anti-IL-22/anti-IL-23 agents. Posology.

Adverse effects. The most notable and grave adverse effects include severe infections, tuberculosis, malignancies, hypersensitivity reactions, headache, fatigue, injection site reaction, joint pain and gastroenteritis [73–75].

Laboratory tests recommended. Physical exam, patient history, complete blood count, liver function, renal function and tuberculosis testing have to be performed before treatment can begin.

Drug interactions. These agents have been noticed to interact with live vaccines. Therefore, it is contraindicated to receive any such vaccines during therapy [3, 73–75].

2.4.3 Ixekizumab, secukinumab and brodalumab

Ixekizumab, secukinumab and brodalumab are systemic anti-IL-17 agents that carry out their roles by expressly inhibiting the IL-17 signalling pathway. Ixekizumab is a humanized IgG4 antibody with a high affinity for IL-17A [76]. Secukinumab is a fully human IgG1 antibody that also blocks IL-17A. Last but not least, brodalumab is a fully human IgG2 antibody that impedes the IL-17 pathway at the receptor level, i.e. by binding to the IL-17RA, a receptor shared by IL-17A and other IL-17 cytokines. For this reason, its effect is broader but more unspecific [77].

Dosage and administration. Ixekizumab, secukinumab and brodalumab are administered as prefilled subcutaneous injections. The induction phase varies from 3 to 12 weeks, followed by the maintenance phase with one or two injections either every second or monthly. **Table 3** illustrates the posology of these therapies [78–80].

Adverse effects. Anti-IL-17 agents may cause serious infections, headache, joint pain, hypertension, diarrhoea, injection site reaction (oedema, pain, erythema, ecchymosis), musculoskeletal pain and hypersensitivity reactions [81].

Laboratory tests recommended. Physical exam, patient history, complete blood count, liver function, renal function and tuberculosis testing must be performed before these therapies as well.

Drug interaction. These agents may interact with drugs that are metabolized by cytochrome P450, e.g. warfarin or cyclosporine [78–80].

Biologic agent	Posology
Ixekizumab	80 mg × 2 at week 0 followed by 80 mg at weeks 2, 4, 6, 8, 10 and 12 and at every 4 weeks afterwards
Secukinumab	150 mg × 2 at weeks 0, 1, 2, 3 and 4 and after the induction phase, 150 mg × 2 is administered once every month
Brodalumab	210 mg × 1 at week 0, 1 and 2, followed by 210 mg × 1 administered every 2 weeks subsequently

Table 3.
Anti-IL-17 agents. Posology.

3. Biological therapies and pregnancy

Despite their presently being no curative remedies for psoriasis, a wide assortment of specific molecular agents exist that are able to ameliorate the symptoms and produce remission. Delivering any of the aforementioned drugs varies primarily on the proficiency of the treating practitioner and only afterwards on the patient's personal choice. It is of utmost importance that women during childbearing age are aware that no studies have been conducted on whether or not these therapies are safe to use while pregnant. Consequently, should any of the biological treatments mentioned except for certolizumab be taken, they must be discontinued prior to conceiving a child. Considering certolizumab, as of writing this chapter, it is ostensibly the only discovered biological agent that fails to cross the maternal-placental barrier, and no adverse or teratogenic consequences were discovered if taken while pregnant [69]. In **Table 4**, we illustrate the minimal time interval suggested between discontinuing the medication and child conception [82].

Therapeutic agent	Contraception
Methotrexate	During pregnancy and at least 3–6 months after
Cyclosporine	Contraception only during the therapy
Acitretin	During pregnancy and at least 3 years after
Fumaric acid esters	During pregnancy and at least 2 weeks after
Apremilast	During pregnancy and 28 days after
Adalimumab	During pregnancy and minimum 5 months after
Etanercept	During pregnancy and 3 weeks after
Ustekinumab	During pregnancy and at least 15 weeks after
Ixekizumab	During pregnancy and at least 6 months after
Secukinumab	During pregnancy and minimum 20 weeks after

Table 4.
Systemic therapy and pregnancy interval.

4. Conclusions

Psoriasis is a debilitating disease with the potential to cause severe psychological damage. In spite of the plentiful advances vis-à-vis treatment, we are still a long way off from obtaining an actual cure. It is crucial to remember that current management strategies only address the symptoms, and not the cause. Therefore, those affected should be closely monitored even in the case of stationary disease or have regression. Moreover, not all therapies correspond to every patient due to possible comorbidities and drug interactions, and thus the notion of a miracle agent in psoriasis appears more and more illusory. This chapter aimed to provide a synopsis of modern treatment options of psoriasis, so that practitioners are sensitized of their uses, contraindications and adverse effects in order to choose the best available strategy.

Acknowledgements

The authors would like to acknowledge the continuous support of Prof. Dr. Remus Orăsan.

Conflict of interest

The authors declare no conflict of interest.

Other declarations

The authors have no further declarations.

Author details

Teodora-Larisa Timis[1*], Daniela-Rodica Mitrea[1] and Ioan-Alexandru Florian[2]

1 Department of Physiology, "Iuliu Hatieganu" University of Medicine and Pharmacy, Cluj-Napoca, Romania

2 Department of Neurosciences, "Iuliu Hatieganu" University of Medicine and Pharmacy, Cluj-Napoca, Romania

*Address all correspondence to: doratimis@gmail.com

IntechOpen

© 2019 The Author(s). Licensee IntechOpen. This chapter is distributed under the terms of the Creative Commons Attribution License (http://creativecommons.org/licenses/by/3.0), which permits unrestricted use, distribution, and reproduction in any medium, provided the original work is properly cited.

References

[1] Institute for Health Metrics and Evaluation (IHME). Global Burden of Disease Study 2010: Results by Cause 1990-2010. Seattle: IHME; 2012

[2] Danielsen K, Olsen AO, Wilsgaard T, Furberg AS. Is the prevalence of psoriasis increasing? A 30–year follow-up of a population-based cohort. The British Journal of Dermatology. 2013;**168**:1303-1310

[3] Martin G, Young M, Aldredge L. Recommendations for initiating systemic therapy in patients with psoriasis. The Journal of Clinical and Aesthetic Dermatology. 2019;**12**(4):13-26

[4] Harden JL, Krueger JG, Bowcock AM. The immunogenetics of psoriasis: A comprehensive review. Journal of Autoimmunity. 2015;**64**:66-73

[5] Rahman M, Alam K, Zaki Ahmad M, et al. Classical to current approach for treatment of psoriasis: A review. Endocrine, Metabolic & Immune Disorders Drug Targets. 2012;**12**:287-302

[6] Cowden A, Van Voorhees AS. Introduction: History of psoriasis and psoriasis therapy. Treatment of Psoriasis. 2008;**1**:1-9. DOI: 10.1007/978-3-7643-7724-3

[7] Brajac I, Gruber F. In: O'Daly J, editor. History of Psoriasis, Psoriasis—A Systemic Disease. IntechOpen; 2012. ISBN: 978-953-51-0281-6. Available from: http://www.intechopen.com/books/psoriasis-asystemic-disease/psoriasis-history-definition-and-treatment-through-centuries

[8] Pusey WA. The History of Dermatology. Springfield, IL: Charles C Thomas; 1933

[9] Glickman FS. Lepra, psora, psoriasis. Journal of the American Academy of Dermatology. 1986;**14**(5 Pt 1):863-866

[10] Willan R. On Cutaneous Diseases. Philadelphia: Kimber and Conrad; 1809

[11] Crissey JT, Parish LC, Shelley WB. The Dermatology and Syphilology of the Nineteenth Century. New York: Praiger Publishers; 1981

[12] Farber EM. Historical commentary. In: Farber EM, Cox AJ, Nall L, Jacobs PH, editors. Psoriasis: Proceedings of the Third International Symposium, Stanford University, 1981. 3rd ed. New York: Grune and Stratton; 1982. pp. 7-11

[13] von Zumbusch LR. Psoriasis und pustuloses exanthem. Archives of Dermatology and Syphilology. 1910;**99**:335-346

[14] Woronoff DL. Die peripheren Veränderungen der Haut um die Effloreszenzen der Psoriasis vulgaris und Syphilis corymbosa. Dermatologische Wochenschrift. 1926;**82**:249-257

[15] Farber EM. History of the treatment of psoriasis. Journal of the American Academy of Dermatology. 1992;**27**(4):640-645. DOI: 10.1016/0190-9622(92)70232-5

[16] Schadler ED, Ortel B, Mehlis SL, et al. Biologics for the primary care physician: Review and treatment of psoriasis. Disease-a-Month. 2019;**65**(3):51-90

[17] Armstrong AW, Schupp C, Wu J, Bebo B. Quality of life and work productivity impairment among psoriasis patients: Findings from the National Psoriasis Foundation survey data 2003-2011. PLoS One. 2012;**7**(12):e52935

[18] Kim J, Krueger JG. The immunopathogenesis of psoriasis. Dermatologic Clinics. 2015;**33**(1):13-23

[19] Gladman DD, Antoni C, Mease P, et al. Psoriatic arthritis: Epidemiology, clinical features, course, and outcome. Annals of the Rheumatic Diseases. 2005;**64**(Suppl 2):ii14-iii7

[20] Nestle FO, Kaplan DH, Barker J. Psoriasis. The New England Journal of Medicine. 2009;**361**(5):496-509

[21] Fitch E, Harper E, Skorcheva I, Kurtz S, Blauvelt A. Pathophysiology of psoriasis: Recent advances on IL-23 and Th17 cytokines. Current Rheumatology Reports. 2007;**9**:461-467

[22] Carvalho AV, Romiti R, Souza CD, et al. Psoriasis comorbidities: Complications and benefits of immunobiological treatment. Anais Brasileiros de Dermatologia. 2016;**91**(6):781-789

[23] Lebwohl MG, Bachelez H, Barker J, et al. Patient perspectives in the management of psoriasis: Results from the population-based Multinational Assessment of Psoriasis and Psoriatic Arthritis Survey. Journal of the American Academy of Dermatology. 2014;**70**(5):871-881

[24] Callis Duffin K, Yeung H, Takeshita J, et al. Patient satisfaction with treatments for moderate-to-severe plaque psoriasis in clinical practice. The British Journal of Dermatology. 2014;**170**(3):672-680

[25] Torsekar R, Gautam MM. Topical therapies in psoriasis. Indian Dermatology Online Journal. 2017;**8**(4):235-245. DOI: 10.4103/2229-5178.209622

[26] Fleischmann HE. Short-contact anthralin therapy for psoriasis. The Western Journal of Medicine. 1987;**147**:461

[27] Goeckerman W. Treatment of psoriasis. Northwest Medicine. 1925;**24**:229-231. [Google Scholar]

[28] Lebwohl M. The role of salicylic acid in the treatment of psoriasis. International Journal of Dermatology. 1999;**38**:16-24

[29] Marsland AM, Griffiths CE. The macrolide immunosuppressants in dermatology: Mechanisms of action. European Journal of Dermatology. 2002;**12**:618-622

[30] Duvic M, Asano AT, Hager C, Mays S. The pathogenesis of psoriasis and the mechanism of action of tazarotene. Journal of the American Academy of Dermatology. 1998;**39** (4 Pt 2):S129-S133

[31] Veraldi S, Caputo R, Pacifico A, Peris K, Soda R, Chimenti S. Short contact therapy with tazarotene in psoriasis vulgaris. Dermatology. 2006;**212**:235-237

[32] Handa S. Newer trends in the management of psoriasis at difficult to treat locations: Scalp, palmoplantar disease and nails. Indian Journal of Dermatology, Venereology and Leprology. 2010;**76**:634-644

[33] Ramsay CA. Management of psoriasis with calcipotriol used as monotherapy. Journal of the American Academy of Dermatology. 1997;**37** (3 Pt 2):S53-S54

[34] Trémezaygues L, Reichrath J. Vitamin D analogs in the treatment of psoriasis: Where are we standing and where will we be going? Dermatoendocrinology. 2011;**3**:180-186

[35] Sabat R, Wolk K, Loyal L, et al. T cell pathology in skin inflammation. Seminars in Immunopathology. 2019;**41**:359-377

[36] Matos TR, Ling TC, Sheth V. Ultraviolet B radiation therapy for psoriasis: Pursuing the optimal regime. Clinics in Dermatology. 2016;**34**:587-593

[37] Kemeny L, Csoma Z, Bagdi E, et al. Targeted phototherapy of plaque-type psoriasis using ultraviolet B-light-emitting diodes. The British Journal of Dermatology. 2010;**163**:167-173

[38] Nishida E, Furuhashi T, Kato H, et al. Successful treatment of psoriasis vulgaris with targeted narrow-band ultraviolet B therapy using a new flat-type fluorescent lamp. Photodermatology, Photoimmunology & Photomedicine. 2011;**27**:248-250

[39] Kemény L, Varga E, Novak Z. Advances in phototherapy for psoriasis and atopic dermatitis. Expert Review of Clinical Immunology. 2019;**15**(11):1205-1214. DOI: 10.1080/1744666X.2020.1672537

[40] Nedelcu RI, Balaban M, Turcu G, et al. Efficacy of methotrexate as anti-inflammatory and anti-proliferative drug in dermatology: Three case reports. Experimental and Therapeutic Medicine. 2019;**18**(2):905-910. DOI: 10.3892/etm.2019.7511

[41] Cheng L. Precision dosage of methotrexate in psoriasis. The British Journal of Dermatology. 2019. DOI: 10.1111/bjd.18273

[42] Bangert CA, Costner MI. Methotrexate in dermatology. Dermatologic Therapy. 2007;**20**:216-228. DOI: 10.1111/j.1529-8019.2007.00135.x

[43] Methotrexate. Fort Lee, NJ: DAVA Pharmaceuticals, Inc.; 2009

[44] Jones KW, Patel SR. A family physician's guide to monitoring methotrexate. American Family Physician. 2000;**62**(7):1607-1612,1614

[45] Neoral. East Hanover, NJ: Novartis Pharmaceuticals Corporation; 2013

[46] Colombo MD, Cassano N, Bellia G, Vena GA. Cyclosporine regimens in plaque psoriasis: An overview with special emphasis on dose, duration, and old and new treatment approaches. Scientific World Journal. 2013;**2013**:805705. DOI: 10.1155/2013/805705

[47] Rosmarin DM, Lebwohl M, Elewski BE, Gottlieb AB. Cyclosporine and psoriasis: 2008 National Psoriasis Foundation Consensus Conference. Journal of the American Academy of Dermatology. 2010;**62**(5):838-853

[48] Maza A, Montaudié H, Sbidian E, et al. Oral cyclosporin in psoriasis: A systematic review on treatment modalities, risk of kidney toxicity and evidence for use in non-plaque psoriasis. Journal of the European Academy of Dermatology and Venereology. 2011;**25**(2):19-27

[49] Clift DE, Thorn RJ, Passarelli EA, et al. Effects of embryonic cyclosporine exposures on brain development and behavior. Behavioural Brain Research. 2015;**282**:117-124. DOI: 10.1016/j.bbr.2015.01.006

[50] Menter A, Korman NJ, Elmets CA, et al. Guidelines of care for the management of psoriasis and psoriatic arthritis: Section 4. Guidelines of care for the management and treatment of psoriasis with traditional systemic agents. Journal of the American Academy of Dermatology. 2009;**61**:451-485

[51] Hsu S, Papp KA, Lebwohl MG, et al. Consensus guidelines for the management of plaque psoriasis. Archives of Dermatology. 2012;**148**:95-102

[52] Schmitt J, Rosumeck S, Thomaschewski G, Sporbeck B, Haufe E, Nast A. Efficacy and safety of systemic treatments for moderate-to-severe psoriasis: Meta-analysis of randomized controlled trials. The British Journal of Dermatology. 2014;**170**:274-303

[53] Soriatane. Research Triangle Park, NC: Stiefel Laboratories Inc.; 2014

[54] Armstrong AW, Aldredge L, Yamauchi PS. Managing patients with psoriasis in the busy clinic: Practical tips for health care practitioners. Journal of Cutaneous Medicine and Surgery. 2016;**20**(3):196-206

[55] Ormerod AD, Mrowietz U. Fumaric acid esters, their place in the treatment of psoriasis. The British Journal of Dermatology. 2004;**150**(4):630-632

[56] Brück J et al. A review of the mechanisms of action of dimethylfumarate (DMF) in the treatment of psoriasis. Experimental Dermatology. 2018;**27**(6):611-624

[57] Skilarence® Summary of Product Characteristics (PDF). Almirall. 2018

[58] Skilarence 120 mg Gastro-resistant Tablets—Summary of Product Characteristics. Electronic Medicines Compendium. 2018. Retrieved 19 July 2018

[59] Schafer P. Apremilast mechanism of action and application to psoriasis and psoriatic arthritis. Biochemical Pharmacology. 2012;**83**(12):1583-1590

[60] Otezla (Prescribing Information). Summit, NJ: Celgene Corporation; 2014. [Retrieved 29 October 2014]

[61] Otezla [Package Insert] June. Summit, NJ: Celgene Corporation; 2017

[62] Stein Gold L, Bagel J, Lebwohl M, Jackson JM, Chen R, Goncalves J, et al. Efficacy and safety of apremilast in systemic- and biologic-naive patients with moderate plaque psoriasis: 52-week results of UNVEIL. Journal of Drugs in Dermatology. 2018;**17**(2):221-228

[63] Gisondi P, Gubinelli E, Cocuroccia B, Girolomoni G. Targeting tumor necrosis factor-alpha in the therapy of psoriasis. Current Drug Targets. Inflammation and Allergy. 2004;**3**(2):175-183

[64] Sbidian E, Chaimani A, Garcia-Doval I, Do G, Hua C, Mazaud C, et al. Systemic pharmacological treatments for chronic plaque psoriasis: A network meta-analysis. Cochrane Database of Systematic Reviews. 2017;(12):Art. No.: CD011535

[65] Remicade (Infliximab). Horsham, PA: Janssen Biotech, Inc.; 2013

[66] Enbrel [Package Insert] November. Thousand Oaks, CA: Immunex Corporation; 2017

[67] Humira (Adalimumab). North Chicago, IL: AbbVie Inc.; 2014

[68] Cimzia [Package Insert] May. Smyrna, GA: UCB, Inc.; 2018

[69] Clowse MEB, Scheuerle AE, Chambers C, et al. Pregnancy outcomes after exposure to certolizumab pegol: Updated results from a pharmacovigilance safety database. Arthritis & Rhematology. 2018;**70**(9):1399-1407. DOI: 10.1002/art.40508

[70] Cingoz O. Ustekinumab. MAbs. 2009;**1**(3):216. DOI: 10.4161/mabs.1.3.8593-221

[71] Al-Salama ZT, Scott LJ. Guselkumab: A review in moderate to severe plaque psoriasis. American Journal of Clinical Dermatology. 2018;**19**(6):907-918. DOI: 10.1007/s40257-018-0406-1

[72] Frampton JE. Tildrakizumab: A review in moderate-to-severe plaque psoriasis. American Journal of Clinical Dermatology. 2019;**20**(2):295-306. DOI: 10.1007/s40257-019-00435-9

[73] Stelara [Prescribing Information]. Horsham, PA: Janssen Biotech, Inc; 2018

[74] Tremfya [Package Insert]. Horsham, PA: Janssen Biotech, Inc.; 2017

[75] Ilumya [Package Insert]. Whitehouse Station, NJ: Merck Sharp & Dohme Corp., a Subsidiary of Merck &Co., Inc.; 2018

[76] Liu L, Lu J, Allan BW, et al. Generation and characterization of ixekizumab, a humanized monoclonal antibody that neutralizes interleukin-17A. Journal of Inflammation Research. 2016;**9**:39-50

[77] Blegvad C, Skov L, Zachariae C. Ixekizumab for the treatment of psoriasis: An update on new data since first approval. Expert Review of Clinical Immunology. 2018;**15**(2):111-121. DOI: 10.1080/1744666X.2019.1559730

[78] Cosentyx [Package Insert]. East Hanover, NJ: Novartis Pharmaceuticals Corporation; 2016

[79] Taltz [Package Insert]. Indianapolis, IN: Eli Lilly and Company; 2017

[80] Siliq [Package Insert]. Bridgewater, NJ: Valeant. Pharmaceuticals North America; 2017

[81] Silfvast-Kaiser A, Paek SY, Menter A. Anti-IL17 therapies for psoriasis. Expert Opinion on Biological Therapy. 2018;**19**(1):45-54. DOI: 10.1080/14712598.2019.1555235

[82] Kraaij G, Balak D, Busard C, Cranenburgh O, Chung Y, Driessen R, et al. Highlights of the updated Dutch evidence- and consensus-based guideline on psoriasis 2017. British Journal of Dermatology. 2019;**180**:31-42. DOI: 10.1111/bjd.17198

Chapter 7

Diagnostic Evaluation of Tuberculosis: Existing Challenges and Merits of Recent Advances

Muhammad Danasabe Isah and Muhammad Aliyu Makusidi

Abstract

Tuberculosis remains a major global public health problem despite the modest infectious disease control efforts. Timely and accurate diagnosis is pivotal to the reduction in tuberculosis related morbidity and mortality. In addition, drug resistant form of tuberculosis is a serious threat to the efforts at tuberculosis control and eradication. Hence; there is the need for efficient methods of *Mycobacterium tuberculosis* infection diagnosis and treatment. There are major advances in the laboratory diagnostic methods for detection of *Mycobacterium tuberculosis* which seeks to complement or replace the existing conventional methods in a view to reduction in under-diagnosis and improved infectious disease management. Chest computer tomographies, Cephid GeneXpert, Line probe are some of the *Mycobacterium tuberculosis* diagnostic advances while chest x-ray, sputum microscopy/culture represent some of the conventional methods of evaluation of both *Mycobacterium tuberculosis* infection and its multi-resistant strain. Intriguingly, the conventional tuberculosis diagnostics though time consuming and inefficient, its use still predominates in high disease burden settings. Meanwhile, the slow transition to use of advanced tuberculosis diagnostic methods seems to have an economic undertone. The seemingly lack of cutting edge advanced *Mycobacterium tuberculosis* diagnostics in high disease burden countries is attributable to their suboptimal health financing model and over reliance on the donor organizations thereby retarding progress in tuberculosis eradication.

Keywords: mycobacteria, evaluation, constraints, advances

1. Introduction

Tuberculosis is a chronic granulomatous bacterial infection with a global occurrence [1–3]. This preventable and curable infectious disease has afflicted man since antiquity [4]. Many parts of the world especially the developing nations are still witnessing a rise in the number of new tuberculosis cases with its attendant consequences [3]. This rising prevalence trend of *Mycobacterium tuberculosis* infection is without prejudice to the strides and efforts in infection control [3].

Estimates have it that every minute someone somewhere gets infected with *Mycobacterium tuberculosis* making it a common globally transmitted disease [5, 6]. Epidemiologically, the World Health Organization (WHO) and other multinational health organization have reported tuberculosis as a worldwide pandemic [3, 7].

IntechOpen

A recent report by WHO revealed a global tuberculosis incidence of 6.3 million for 2016 reflecting a rise from the preceding year [3]. In the same vein, sub Saharan Africa has a substantial burden of tuberculosis related morbidity and mortality as reported in the 2016 WHO global tuberculosis report [3].

The current epidemiological profile of tuberculosis in Sub-Saharan Africa seems to have an established association of the disease with poverty and social deprivation [3, 5, 8]. Similarly, the burden of tuberculosis remains an obstacle to socioeconomic development with a staggering direct and indirect cost of health financing [3, 9, 10]. The relationship between tuberculosis and social deprivation in addition to the adverse socioeconomic developmental effect of tuberculosis creates a vicious cycle of disease, poverty and poor productivity among the most disadvantaged in the society.

Mycobacterium tuberculosis is the causative organism of tuberculosis which was discovered by Robert Koch [11]. This granuloma forming microorganism is well adapted to live in a man and cause disease under favorable condition(s). In the same token, *Mycobacterium tuberculosis* is ubiquitous and has some unique features in its genetic makeup and cell wall constituents that not only distinct it from other organisms but also confers it with the strength of survival under harsh and stressful conditions [12, 13].

The *Mycobacterium tuberculosis* genome is composed of insertion sequences (IS) and phages which serve as unique features for its identification and speciation [12]. The type of IS that is abundant in *Mycobacterium tuberculosis* is IS6110 [12]. The knowledge of *Mycobacterium tuberculosis* genome is used in assessment of rate of transmission, identification of a regional circulating strain and detection of trans-border spread of the disease.

The main stay of *Mycobacterium tuberculosis* diagnosis has been the sputum microscopy (Ziehl Neelsen) and the solid media culture (Lowestein-Jensen medium) [14]. Although, these conventional methods of *Mycobacterium tuberculosis* identification and isolation are still in use, newer methods of tuberculosis diagnostics which include Ampiclor *M. tuberculosis* PCR test and Cephid GeneXpert is fast gaining relevance and acceptance [15, 16]. The merits of use of molecular and immunological techniques cannot be overemphasized in view of its additional benefit of infectious organism speciation, isolate antimicrobial sensitivity and detection of specific mutations that confer drug resistance (i.e., rpoB and KatG mutation) [15, 16]. The acquisition and deployment of molecular tuberculosis diagnostics in priority high disease burden areas would eventually increase rate of *Mycobacterium tuberculosis* infection identification. This is predicated on the fact that early detection and treatment of smear positive tuberculosis is attributed to improved cure rate [15].

2. Aim and objectives

This chapter is an exploratory study of existing tuberculosis diagnostics aimed at highlighting the conventional and advanced methods of *Mycobacterium tuberculosis* evaluation. The objective is to identify suitable and efficient method(s) of tuberculosis detection by way of profiling their merits and demerits.

3. Methods

This chapter is a descriptive research on the evolutionary trend of tuberculosis diagnosis. Available literature would be used to identify existing methods of *Mycobacterium tuberculosis* detection. A comparative analysis between the merits and demerits of old conventional and advanced molecular/immunological methods would be carried out to ascertain what best serve the purpose of prompt and efficient detection of *Mycobacterium tuberculosis* infection.

4. Literature review

4.1 Global burden of tuberculosis

Mycobacterium tuberculosis infection remains a significant public health challenge despite the modest achievements in its control at the global, regional and country levels [3]. The alarming global prevalence rate of *Mycobacterium tuberculosis* infection has been put at one-third of the world population [1, 3]. Sub-Saharan Africa, South East Asia, and West Pacific region is home to most of the 22 countries highly burdened by tuberculosis, and this ranking seldom change [3, 17].

World Health Organization reported that 6.3 million cases of tuberculosis were notified in 2016 which might be under-estimation owing to the non-health seeking behavior and poor documentation in some regions [3]. This tuberculosis epidemiological pattern calls for sustained surveillance and prompt treatment to improve the disease related morbidity and mortality [3].

The rising number of drug-resistant form of tuberculosis poses an additional challenge on the inadequate resources allocated to healthcare delivery. In the year 2015, over 100 countries reported extensively drug-resistant tuberculosis [2]. Estimates by the WHO revealed that 490,000 individual developed multidrug-resistant tuberculosis in the year 2016 and only a fraction received treatment [3]. The threat of drug-resistant tuberculosis as affirmed by 2016 global report on tuberculosis may possibly be a consequence of inappropriate anti-tuberculosis medication use [3]. This emerging menace of drug resistant tuberculosis if not properly managed could retard the progress made in the fight against tuberculosis.

The global distribution of tuberculosis infection is in close association with poverty, immunosuppression and social deprivation [3, 5, 8, 17]. Sub Saharan Africa has the world highest tuberculosis incidence of 356 per 100,000 populations per year [2, 3]. Similarly, the social and clinical determinants of tuberculosis which include HIV infection, diabetes mellitus, under-nutrition, migration and smoking have been reported to preferentially afflict the young adult population [3, 5]. Nevertheless, tuberculosis infection generally has no age, gender, racial or regional bias.

Mycobacteria consist of different pathogenic and saprophytic mycobacteria species that are isolated from humans and the general environment [18, 19]. The two broad groups of mycobacteria which are tuberculous and non-tuberculous mycobacteria share some features but are largely distinguishable by molecular analysis and the utilization of some microbiological test which include niacin reduction test, nitrate test, and urease test [18, 19]. Lack of identification of the species of mycobacteria infection from the outset has a clinical, management and prognostic implication. The importance of mycobacteria speciation lie in their differing epidemiology, response to anti-tuberculosis, course of disease and long term consequences [18, 19].

4.2 Pulmonary and extra-pulmonary tuberculosis

Literally, tuberculosis could affect any organ system of the body and clinical presentation depends on the site of involvement. The human host immune system influences the clinical pattern of tuberculosis presentation. Tuberculosis is generally described as pulmonary if it involves the lungs and extra-pulmonary when there is involvement of other body parts excluding the lungs [8, 20]. This disease has also been described as latent tuberculosis and active/open tuberculosis.

The initial *Mycobacterium tuberculosis* infection could be dormant and symptomless (latent tuberculosis) or it could be symptomatic (progressive primary tuberculosis) manifesting commonly as miliary tuberculosis, primary tuberculous pneumonia, and tuberculous meningitis [21].

Research has shown that 95% of primary *Mycobacterium tuberculosis* infection is contained and represented as Ghon focus on the chest radiograph [21, 22]. Post-primary tuberculosis is the most frequent mode of presentation of pulmonary *Mycobacterium tuberculosis* infection [21, 22]. This form of tuberculosis could result from an endogenous reactivation of the dormant bacilli from the primary infection or a reinfection with *Mycobacterium tuberculosis*.

Clinical manifestations of tuberculosis are body site-specific but may be subclinical thereby posing a diagnostic challenge with frequent missed clinical cases. Commonly, patients with tuberculosis have constitutional symptoms in addition to body site specific symptom(s) [8, 23–25]. The diagnostic challenge of tuberculosis is frequently observed among children and the elderly probably due to their unique immune constitution and the nature of their airway defense mechanism [22, 25, 26].

Clinical manifestation of pulmonary tuberculosis serves as a prototype of *Mycobacterium tuberculosis* infection with specific and non-specific clinical presentations. Cough is the predominant symptom of pulmonary tuberculosis [23–25]. Chronic cough lasting for at least 2 weeks has been used as a flag off symptom for initiating tuberculosis evaluation among individuals at the community level [3]. Difficulty in breathing, chest pain, and chest deformity could be addition complaints by the patients with pulmonary tuberculosis [23–25].

The physical examination equally poses an additional diagnostic challenge as clinical findings could be non-specific and unhelpful in diagnosis. Pulmonary tuberculosis patients usually have respiratory system specific clinical signs of disease or complication that include crepitation, bronchial breath sound, amphoric adventitious sound and pleural rub [23–25]. Noteworthy is the clinical manifestation of extensive lung destruction by way of fibrosis and contraction of lung volume [27].

4.3 Tuberculosis detection methods

4.3.1 Sputum microscopy/culture

The goal of investigation is to make a speedy, definite and accurate diagnosis of *Mycobacterium tuberculosis* infection and to identify complication(s) of the disease. The advances in tuberculosis investigation have provided increased sensitivity and have assisted in improving transit time to diagnosis [28, 29].

Sputum microscopy (Ziehl Neelsen) is a common method for microbiological profiling of *Mycobacterium tuberculosis* infection, especially in resource-limited countries [14, 28]. The fluorescence microscopy for *Mycobacterium tuberculosis* though not readily available is an alternative to sputum microscopy (Ziehl Neelsen) [30]. Both investigations use dye for staining but additionally, the fluorescence microscopy requires the light-emitting diodes (LED) to visualize *Mycobacterium tuberculosis* in sputum sample.

Although, sputum microscopy is cheap and can be rapidly performed, it is operator dependent and its cost-effectiveness is marred by a decreased sensitivity in pauci-bacillary states [15]. This diagnostic limitation has made extra-pulmonary tuberculosis difficult to diagnose. The rate of false-positive results and inter-operator differences in reportage of sputum microscopy has also compelled the need to recognize molecular based investigation (Cephid GeneXpert) as the first line investigation for tuberculosis [15, 31]. Sputum microscopy is likely to continuously be a cornerstone investigation in the evaluation of tuberculosis patient in the resource constraint nations going by its cost-effectiveness. Hence, the need to improve its operational capacity by way of research and development.

Sputum culture for *Mycobacterium tuberculosis* represents an improvement well and above microscopy, making it a definitive investigation of choice for the isolation and identification of the infective organism [28–30]. Sputum culture has a better sensitivity and specificity when compared with sputum microscopy [15, 31]. In view of this superiority, clinicians are advised to obtain culture confirmation of tuberculosis where feasible.

Mycobacteria solid culture media which is typified by Lowenstein, Stonebrink, or Ogawa medium is the predominant and sometimes the only form of culture used in evaluation of tuberculosis [15, 32]. This mycobacteria culture is cheap, limits contamination but slow taking about 4–8 weeks to detection of culture growth. The merits of mycobacteria solid media culture is beclouded by the long transition to diagnosis which is inimical to tuberculosis control because it delays commencement of treatment. In contrast, liquid media which is represented by Bacteria Mycobacterial Growth Indicator Tube 960 and MB/Bact Alert 10 3D is more sensitive, faster in detection of growth and the gold standard for mycobacteria isolation [15]. The study by Munyati et al., estimated cost of mycobacteria liquid culture (1–3 culture) to be in the range of $53–$163 [32]. By this estimated cost it is considered to be impracticable to recommend mycobacteria liquid media culture in resource limited setting despite its cost-effectiveness in *Mycobacterium tuberculosis* infection detection and isolation. The cost of procurement and maintenance of mycobacteria liquid media culture may have informed the reason for its low availability and utilization.

4.3.2 Radiologic study

Radiographic profiling for tuberculosis is an indispensable investigation in the evaluation of infected patients. This investigative modality had a remarkable evolution from the use of the x-rays to the use of advanced imaging modalities which include the computer tomographic scan thereby upping the radiographic sensitivity and specificity [25, 30].

A normal x-ray does not rule out tuberculosis, and no radiological finding is a sine qua non for tuberculosis. This reality poses a diagnostic challenge for health care providers especially in the evaluation of tuberculosis among the immune-compromised. The x-ray imaging findings are predominantly abnormal in pulmonary tuberculosis among the immune-competent [30, 33]. The upper zone and apical lobe of the lower zone of the lungs are areas of predilection in pulmonary tuberculosis [30]. In pulmonary tuberculosis, the commonest x-ray manifestation is parenchyma involvement which is depicted by linear opacities, cavitations and military shadows [15]. Pleural effusion, pleural thickening, lymphadenopathy, and tuberculoma are the other extra-pulmonary manifestations that could be evident on the chest radiographic examination.

Following chronic inflammation from *Mycobacterium tuberculosis* infection, healing leaves behind nodules and parenchymal scarring. This is the radiologist nightmare and a diagnostic challenge because residual x-ray findings represent a stable disease but does not rule out active tuberculosis. In addition, atypical findings on radiographs of immune-compromised individuals may lead to misdiagnosis of *Mycobacterium tuberculosis* infection.

Chest computer tomography (CT) provides a diagnostic advantage in detecting fine and equivocal lesions among tuberculosis patients when compared with x-ray films [15]. The findings on chest CT which could represent an active disease or disease complications include features suggestive of consolidation, fibrosis, cavitations and honey combing [15]. Similarly, the chest CT provides a clearer view of extra-pulmonary involvement of *Mycobacterium tuberculosis* infection. For example a "tree in bud" appearance on chest CT sufficiently represents active disease which may not be discernible on x-ray films [15]. Despite, the added advantage of chest CT over chest x-ray, microbiological test for *Mycobacterium tuberculosis* is essential for a definitive diagnosis.

4.3.3 Molecular methods

Tuberculin skin test for the latent tuberculosis is an ancient molecular investigation that still reserves a place in clinical practice [30]. A major drawback of tuberculin skin test is its inability to differentiate the latent tuberculosis from an active disease. This diagnostic drawback has a therapeutic and prognostic implication. Line probe assay and Cephid GeneXpert System are the other advanced molecular investigations that have enabled detection of drug resistant tuberculosis [30]. Cephid GeneXpert System has been recommended as the first choice tuberculosis investigation especially among suspected cases of multidrug resistant disease [34, 35]. This decision may have been predicated on the suitability of Cephid GeneXpert System for use in resource limited environment due to its adequate sensitivity, specificity and the minimal technical knowhow for its operation [34, 35]. However, this guideline should be cautiously recommended for developing nations because they may not cope with its financial implication.

Lipoarabinomannan (LAM) assay in urine has been commercially available for over 20 years but its deployment for use in tuberculosis diagnostics is slow [36]. This molecular investigation is a point-of-care assay that enables detection of LAM which is a mycobacterial cell wall glycolipid antigen [36, 37]. Lipoarabinomannan assay in urine has enabled diagnosis of disseminated tuberculosis especially in pauci-bacillary state and among HIV patients. A meta-analytic study has reported a sub-optimal sensitivity for LAM assay in urine [38]. However, subsequent improvement in LAM assay in urine by way of development of strip test version of this molecular investigation improved its sensitivity, specificity and cost-effectiveness.

4.3.4 Immunological methods

Immunological investigations for active tuberculosis include nucleic acid amplification tests and bacteriophage-based tests. These immunological investigations have allowed detection of nucleic acid sequence of *Mycobacterium tuberculosis* and assisted in genetic finger typing [28–30]. In furtherance, immunological methods of *Mycobacterium tuberculosis* diagnosis provide an opportunity for the infective organism speciation (MicroSeq 500 system, AccuProbe assay) and drug sensitivity test [30]. Worthy of mention in the deployment of immunological investigation for multidrug resistance evaluation are assessment of the rpoB gene mutation for rifampicin resistance, the inhA gene and the katG gene mutation for low and high level isoniazid resistance, respectively [30, 39].

In contrast to smear microscopy/culture, nucleic acid amplification test has a greater positive predictive value (>95%), increase specificity and ability for rapid confirmation of infection [15]. Nevertheless, the smear microscopy/culture still has relevance in modern clinical practice because of its high sensitivity and utility when drug sensitivity test of second line anti-tuberculosis is required [15].

5. Conclusion

In conclusion, there is need to complement and replace where necessary the conventional tuberculosis diagnostics with advanced cutting-edge microbiological, imaging, molecular and immunologic investigations for prompt and adequate diagnosis. The diagnostic and therapeutic advantages of advanced methods of mycobacteria detection call for its speedy deployment to priority areas to enhance accuracy and efficiency of clinical evaluation. The cost of procurement and maintenance of this advanced methods of tuberculosis diagnosis maybe beyond the reach of the health care systems of nations with high burden by tuberculosis. Hence, the reason why donor funding is crucial in provision and maintenance of advanced molecular and immunological tuberculosis diagnostics in high disease burden areas especially in sub-Saharan Africa [40, 41].

Author details

Muhammad Danasabe Isah* and Muhammad Aliyu Makusidi
Usmanu Danfodiyo University, Sokoto, Nigeria

*Address all correspondence to: muzaifa2007@gmail.com

IntechOpen

© 2019 The Author(s). Licensee IntechOpen. This chapter is distributed under the terms of the Creative Commons Attribution License (http://creativecommons.org/licenses/by/3.0), which permits unrestricted use, distribution, and reproduction in any medium, provided the original work is properly cited. (cc) BY

References

[1] World Health Organization Fact Sheet on Tuberculosis. 2015. Available from: http://www.who.int/mediacentre/factsheets/fs104/en/ [Accessed: 14 January 2016]

[2] World Health Organization Global Tuberculosis Report. Geneva: WHO; 2016. Available from: http://apps.who.int/iris/bitstream/10665/250441/1/9789241565394-eng.pdf?ua=1 [Accessed: 08 November 2016]

[3] World Health Organization Global Tuberculosis Report. Geneva: WHO; 2017. Available from: http://www.who.int/tb/publications/global_report/gtbr2016_executive_summary.pdf [Accessed: 28 November 2017]

[4] Holloway KL, Henneberg RJ, de Barros Lopes M, Henneberg M. Evolution of human tuberculosis: A systematic review and meta-analysis of paleopathological evidence. Homo. 2011;**62**:402-458

[5] Philippe G, Charalambos S, Katherine F, Mario R. Global epidemiology of tuberculosis. Cold Spring Harbor Perspectives in Medicine. 2015;**5**

[6] Giorgia S, Alberto R, Alberto M, Mario CR. Tuberculosis: Epidemiology and control. Mediterranean Journal of Hematology and Infectious Diseases. 2014;**6**(1):e2014070. DOI: 10.4084/MJHID.2014.070

[7] Center for Diseases Control and Prevention. Tuberculosis: Data and Statistics. 2017. Available from: https://www.cdc.gov/tb/statistics/default.htm [Accessed: 10 November 2017]

[8] Siddaraya H, Sanganna LL. Study of sociodemographic and clinical features of tuberculosis cases in HIV patients. National Journal of Integrated Research in Medicine. 2016;7(4):28-32

[9] Nicola F, Anna V, Susan C, Lucy C, Gavin C, Edina S. The economic burden of TB diagnosis and treatment in South Africa. Social Science and Medicine. 2015;**130**:42-50

[10] Andreas F, Ole H, Christian W, Anders L, Rikke I, Jakob K, et al. The economic burden of tuberculosis in Denmark 1998–2010. Cost analysis in patients and their spouses. International Journal of Infectious Diseases. 2015;**32**:183-190

[11] Gursimrat KS. Tuberculosis: Current situation, challenges and overview of its control programs in India. Journal of Global Infectious Diseases. 2011;**3**(2):143-150

[12] Anamika G, Savita K, Nalin R, Shampa A. A study of mycobacterium tuberculosis genotypic diversity and drug resistance mutations in Varanasi, North India. The Indian Journal of Medical Research. 2014;**139**(6):892-902

[13] Erik CH, Eric JR. Bacterial growth and cell division: A mycobacterial perspective. Microbiology and Molecular Biology Reviews. 2008;**72**(1):126-156

[14] Linda MP, Ákos S, Cristina G, Evan L, Paramasivan CN, Alash'le A, et al. Laboratory diagnosis of tuberculosis in resource-poor countries: Challenges and opportunities. Clinical Microbiology Reviews. 2011;**24**(2):314-350

[15] Yon JR. Diagnosis of pulmonary tuberculosis: Recent advances and diagnostic algorithms. Tuberculosis Respiratory Disease. 2015;**78**(2):64-71

[16] Mochammad H, Sultan AR. Tuberculosis—Current Issues in Diagnosis and Management. 2018. Available from: http://www.intechopen.com/books/tuberculosis-current-issues-indiagnosis-and-management [Accessed: 20 March 2018]

[17] Christopher D. Global epidemiology of tuberculosis. Lancet. 2006;**367**(9514): 938-940

[18] Roland D, Josephine J, Niklas L, Michael L, Albert N, Klaus FR, et al. Burden of non-tuberculous mycobacterial pulmonary disease in Germany. European Respiratory Journal. 2017;**49**:1602109. DOI: 10.1183/13993003.02109-2016

[19] Margaret MJ, John AO. Nontuberculous mycobacterial pulmonary infections. Journal of Thoracic Disease. 2014;**6**(3):210-220

[20] Rajiv CM, Joy SM. Tuberculosis in otorhinolaryngology: Clinical presentation and diagnostic challenges. International Journal of Otolaryngology. 2011;**2011**:4. DOI: 10.1155/2011/686894. Article ID 686894

[21] Hee JY, Young GS, Woo IP, Jae PC, Kyung HC, June MK. Clinical manifestations and diagnosis of extra-pulmonary tuberculosis. Yonsei Medical Journal. 2004;**45**(3):453-461

[22] Andrea TC, Jeffrey RS. Clinical manifestations of tuberculosis in children. Paediatric Respiratory Reviews. 2007;**8**(2):107-117

[23] Barman TK, Roy S, Hossain MA, Bhuiyan GR, Abedin S. Clinical presentation of adult pulmonary tuberculosis (PTB): A study of 103 cases from a tertiary care hospital. Mymensingh Medical Journal. 2017; **26**(2):235-240

[24] Bayat S, Gol-Mohamadi A, Sarbazi MR, Safaee A, Farsar AR, et al. A seven year retrospective study on epidemiology and clinical characteristics of tuberculosis in Iran. Archives of Clinical Infectious Diseases. 2013;**8**(2): ee14505. DOI: 10.5812/archcid.14505

[25] Yong SK, Su YC, In JO, Kyu Sik K, Kim YI, Sung CL, et al. Clinical characteristics and treatment outcomes of tuberculosis in the elderly: A case control study. BMC Infectious Diseases. 2013;**13**:121

[26] Susanna E, Claudia T, Samantha B. Tuberculosis in children. Mediterranean Journal of Hematology and Infectious Diseases. 2013;**5**(1):e2013064

[27] Diego VP, Oscar P, Esther P, Jordi A. Radiological findings of unilateral tuberculous lung destruction. Insights Imaging. 2017;**8**(2):271-277

[28] James JD, Jeffrey RS, Paula AR. Laboratory diagnosis of mycobacterium tuberculosis infection and disease in children. Journal of Clinical Microbiology. 2016;**54**(6):1434-1441

[29] Stephen DL. Advances in diagnostic assays for tuberculosis. Cold Spring Harbor Perspectives in Medicine. 2015; **5**(12):a017806

[30] Jindal SK, Shankar PS, Raoof S, Gupta D, Aggarwal AN, Agarwal R. Handbook of Pulmonary and Critical Care Medicine. 1st ed. India: Jaypee Brothers Medical Publishers (P) Ltd; 2012. ISBN 978-93-5025-707-4

[31] Matthew DE, Neil WS, Amy LD, Stanley B, William NR, Bruce H. Time to detection of *Mycobacterium tuberculosis* in sputum culture correlates with outcome in patients receiving treatment for pulmonary tuberculosis. Chest. 1998;**113**(2):379-386

[32] Munyati SS, Dhoba T, Makanza ED, Mungofa S, Wellington M, Mutsvangwa J, et al. Chronic cough in primary health care attendees, Harare, Zimbabwe: Diagnosis and impact of HIV infection. Clinical Infectious Diseases. 2005;**40**: 1818-1827

[33] Aline B, Guilherme JS, Rosemeri MS. Clinical, radiological, and laboratory characteristics in pulmonary tuberculosis patients: Comparative

study of HIV-positive and HIV-negative inpatients at a referral hospital. Jornal Brasileiro de Pneumologia. Nov-Dec 2011; **37**(6):768-775

[34] Monika A, Ashish B, Vinay B, Sarjana D. Comparative study of GeneXpert with ZN stain and culture in samples of suspected pulmonary tuberculosis. Journal of Clinical and Diagnostic Research. 2016;**10**(5):DC09-DC12

[35] Ravdeep K, Kavita K, Jitendar KS, Satyanarayana MV, Amit D. Diagnostic accuracy of Xpert test in tuberculosis detection: A systematic review and meta-analysis. Journal of Global Infectious Diseases. 2016;**8**(1):32-40

[36] Stephen DL, Ankur G. Detection of lipoarabinomannan (LAM) in urine is indicative of disseminated TB with renal involvement in patients living with HIV and advanced immunodeficiency: Evidence and implications. Transactions of the Royal Society of Tropical Medicine and Hygiene. 2016;**110**(3): 180-185

[37] Stephen DL, Kerkhoff AD, Vogt M, Wood R. Diagnostic accuracy of a low-cost, urine antigen, point-of-care screening assay for HIV-associated pulmonary tuberculosis before antiretroviral therapy: A descriptive study. The Lancet Infectious Diseases. 2012;**12**(3):201-209

[38] Minion j l E, Talbot E, Dheda K, Pai M, Menzies D. Diagnosing tuberculosis with urine lipoarabinomannan: Systemic review and meta-analysis. The European Respiratory Journal. 2011;**38**: 1398-1405

[39] Jagielski T, Grzeszczuk M, Kamiński M, Roeske K, Napiórkowska A, Stachowiak R, et al. Identification and analysis of mutations in the katG gene in multidrug-resistant mycobacterium tuberculosis clinical isolates. Pneumonologia i Alergologia Polska. 2013;**81**(4):298-307

[40] Mike F. 2016 Report on Tuberculosis Research Funding Trends 2005–2015. 2018. Available from: www.treatmentactiongroup.org/sites/default/files/TB_FUNDING_2016_WEB.pdf [Accessed: 23 March 2018]

[41] Katherine F, Christopher F, Andrea P, Mario R. Domestic and donor financing for tuberculosis care and control in low-income and middle-income countries: An analysis of trends, 2002–2011, and requirements to meet 2015 targets. The Lancet. 2013;**1**(2): e105-e115

Chapter 8

Loss to Follow-Up (LTFU) during Tuberculosis Treatment

Kyaw San Lin

Abstract

Loss to follow-up (LTFU) is a serious issue in the field of tuberculosis (TB) since it can lead to TB outbreaks and drug resistance. The proportion of LTFU patients differs among different countries, regions, year, and institutions. In some countries, the number of patients that were LTFU nearly reaches half of the total patients. Underlying factors such as age, gender, education, residence, financial factors, migration, and social stigma are discussed in this chapter. These factors should always be taken into consideration whenever a treatment program is designed. Suggestions have been made regarding some interventions that could potentially solve the problem of LTFU. With these points in mind, an ambitious approach should be taken to reduce the number of LTFU patients up to zero.

Keywords: tuberculosis, TB, loss to follow-up, LTFU, default

1. Introduction

Tuberculosis (TB) is a disease, which requires more than just biomedical treatment. WHO-recommended standard TB treatment requires a minimum duration of 6 months. The patients have to regularly take treatment without interruption to get a cure. However, discontinuation of treatment because of loss to follow-up (LTFU) is a significant problem, especially among patients suffering from multidrug-resistant tuberculosis (MDR-TB), requiring urgent attention. The proportions of LTFU and its associated factors differ among various countries. A clear understanding of these underlying causes is essential for the success and effectiveness of the National Tuberculosis Program (NTP) of every nation. Hence, appropriate measures targeting LTFU are needed to achieve the goals of the NTP.

2. Definition

In 2012, a large group of researchers from Africa, Asia, America, Europe, and the Pacific suggested that the term 'defaulter' is inappropriate for the patient [1]. Instead, they recommended using the term 'person lost to follow-up' to become more patient-centered. In 2013, the WHO decided to use the term 'loss to follow-up' instead of 'defaulter' for reporting treatment outcomes because the former is less judgmental [2]. They defined LTFU as "A TB patient who did not start treatment or whose treatment was interrupted for 2 consecutive months or more." Since then, several papers have started reporting according to this new term and definition [3–10].

IntechOpen

3. The problem of LTFU

The patients who were LTFU have not completed the treatment regime. This can cause serious public health problems because these patients are at higher risk of drug resistance [11]. They continue to spread the potentially resistant bacilli to the public, infecting the public. This has been proved in a Bayesian mapping where LTFU has served as an important indicator for the distribution of TB patients [12]. Therefore, LTFU should be one of our primary concerns in the battle against TB.

Even just a single case of LTFU could cause an outbreak of TB, as observed in countries with low incidence such as Norway [13, 14], USA [15], and Austria [16]. In such outbreaks, the index cases are mostly immigrants, spreading the infection to their families, friends, and other social networks. To further visualize this problem, we need to look into the proportion of LTFU among different countries in the world.

4. Proportion of LTFU

The proportion of LTFU varies considerably among different countries, different types of TB, and different patient populations. It has been studied extensively and was found to be ranging from 2.5 to 44.9% [17–23]. A very high proportion (44.9%) of the patients were LTFU in rural northern Mozambique revealing that LTFU is a very serious problem [19]. In addition, systematic reviews and meta-analyses have estimated the mean proportion of multidrug-resistant TB patients who were LTFU. A 2009 systematic review of MDR-TB patients has found that this proportion is 12% [24]. Another 2009 systematic review also found a similar proportion of 13% [25]. However, a 2012 individual patient data meta-analysis found a higher proportion of 23% [26]. A rough literature review has revealed that the proportion of MDR TB patients who were LTFU ranges from 2.2 to 47% [27–43]. The figures vary vastly among different years, countries, and institutions, suggesting that the underlying factors responsible for these variations should be studied carefully.

However, few studies have reported on the proportion of LTFU among patients with extra-pulmonary TB. According to a French study, this proportion was 25% among lymph node TB patients [44]. Another study from Gabon reported that the proportion among cervical lymph node TB patients was 24.3% [45]. In India, among the miliary tuberculosis patients presenting with neurological manifestations, the proportion was 10% [46]. However, in Saudi Arabia, the proportion among CNS tuberculoma patients was reported to be 25.8% [47].

Another area of interest is latent TB since developed countries such as the USA and the UK are giving much attention to latent TB and its LTFU rate. Studies from the USA reported proportions ranging from 12 to 35.6% [48, 49]. In the UK, this proportion is 22.8% [50], and in Switzerland, 11% [51].

Attention should also be paid toward LTFU among certain special populations. The proportion of LTFU among childhood TB patients ranges from 4 to 37% [52–57]. Among the children with drug-resistant TB, it ranges from 5 to 19.09% [58–60]. These figures are much similar to those of the adult population. On the other hand, researchers from Côte d'Ivoire found out that the proportion of LTFU was rising among the elderly TB patients [61]. This is an area that researchers should explore more in the future.

We should not forget about our fellow healthcare workers since LTFU could lead to serious problems in the healthcare service setting. They are expected to have low rates of LTFU because of the medical knowledge they possess. Fortunately, a study from Morocco confirmed that the proportion of LTFU among healthcare workers in the public sector was only 0.8% [62]. However, many studies need to be done to explore this area of study.

Other populations of interest are prisoners and migrants. Northern Ethiopian prisons reported a low LTFU proportion of only 2.5% [63], which is an excellent result. In contrast, among the Ugandan prison inmates, 43% were LTFU and the odds are greater among the transferred prisoners [64]. On the other hand, researchers from the USA found out that 25.8% of the cases in a public health intervention were LTFU, and they were mainly undocumented migrants [65]. In such countries, as discussed above, even a single case of LTFU can cause an outbreak of TB. The same problem is arising in Australia where all of the detained illegal foreign fishermen were LTFU [66]. They concluded that

"Treatment completion in illegal foreign fishermen may be as low as zero; deporting fishermen before curative treatment is completed undermines TB control efforts and may lead to an emergence of drug resistance and an increased burden of active TB disease in our region."

This is an area of concern that needs urgent measures. On the other hand, the International Organization of Migration is achieving great results among Vietnamese immigrants [67]. Only 7% of the MDR-TB patients from these migrants were LTFU. It is likely that such 'international intergovernmental' effort is necessary to tackle the problem of LTFU among the migrants since individual governments are facing difficulties handling this problem.

5. Factors associated with LTFU

5.1 Individual factors

Individual factors play a role in the process of being LTFU from treatment. Sometimes, the results may contradict between different studies, probably due to the cultural, social, and other variations of the study settings.

Among the various sociodemographic characteristics, age is a recognized factor associated with LTFU. Studies from India, Brazil, and China revealed that elderly patients have higher LTFU [4, 68–70], whereas studies from Norway, Botswana, and South Africa suggested that adolescents have significant risk [8, 30, 71]. One study from the UK even suggested a wider range of age of 15–44 years as a high-risk group for LTFU [11]. Regarding gender, studies uniformly suggest that higher LTFU was found in males, as seen in Kenya, Ethiopia, Georgia, and Uzbekistan [7, 18, 41, 72].

Residence plays a role in the mechanism of LTFU. In Pakistan, the rural residence is associated with LTFU [73], whereas in Uzbekistan, the urban residence is associated with LTFU [18]. This may be caused by access to the treatment center since being far from the treatment center is also associated with LTFU [74]. Transportation should be improved to increase accessibility toward the treatment center. Alternatively, they could be built in the hard-to-reach areas. Both approaches include challenges, and ultimately, these challenges may be what cause LTFU. Further discussion regarding different providers will be given in the next section.

Education plays a role in the development of LTFU. Brazilian researchers have found out that less than 8 years of schooling increases the risk of LTFU [4]. In addition, scarce TB knowledge is a risk factor for LTFU [75], and better TB knowledge a protective factor [5]. Therefore, health education and proper counseling should always be at the heart of every anti-TB treatment program.

Financial factors should also be considered while giving treatment, and programs without such considerations will likely to result in high LTFU. A study from

Uzbekistan found that joblessness contributes toward LTFU [18]. This is confirmed by a study from China which found that pre-school children, unemployed laborers, and retirees have a higher rate of LTFU [76]. Patients with low income have financial constraints to complete treatment leading to LTFU as seen in India [77], a lower middle-income country. A similar phenomenon has been observed in South Korea, a high-income country [78]. Even in the USA, it was found that homelessness is associated with LTFU [79, 80], which might be due to low income. Therefore, regardless of the country, patients with low income still have barriers against treatment completion.

LTFU is also associated with alcohol abuse, tobacco use, smoking, and illicit drug use. Association between alcoholism and LTFU was observed in India [77], Philippines [5], and Congo [74], tobacco use in Georgia [41], smoking in Brazil [75], and illicit drug use in Norway [30], Georgia [41], and the UK [81]. Therefore, before initiating treatment, personal history should be carefully taken to find out these risk factors, and special attention should be given to such patients.

There are also certain disease-specific factors that are associated with LTFU. Those who were previously LTFU tend to be LTFU again. This was confirmed by studies conducted in Brazil [4], Kenya [7], Uzbekistan [18], and Korea [78]. Caution should be taken while planning treatment for such patients. Studies from Nigeria and Ethiopia both point out that smear-negative TB patients were more likely to be LTFU [72, 82]. However, the opposite was observed in the UK where smear-positive pulmonary TB patients were more likely to be LTFU [11]. Researchers also found that patients with extrapulmonary TB were more likely to be LTFU [71, 83]. Co-morbid diseases such as diabetes mellitus and human immunodeficiency virus (HIV) infection also cause hindrance against TB treatment conditions [7, 71, 84].

5.2 Treatment support services

The treatment providers should give support to the patients since a perceived lack of provider support is a barrier to regular follow-up [77], and receiving any type of assistance and support from the providers can protect against LTFU [5]. They need to build up trust [5] from the patients. An intervention program targeting these factors will be described later in the chapter. Lastly, the timing of the treatment services should be flexible according to the needs of the patients [77], but this may not be an easy task to implement.

5.3 Diagnosis and treatment

The timing of the treatment is important since those who initiate the treatment late (beyond and within 30 days of onset) are more likely to be LTFU [85]. Those who initiate it late may not have enough motivation, will, or knowledge to continue taking treatment until they are cured. Moreover, the timing of treatment interruption is found to be the most important during the intensive phase [7]. This stage should be particularly targeted while conducting interventions against LTFU.

Different providers have different abilities to retain the patients. In Korea, patients treated by a non-pulmonologist were found to be more likely to default from TB treatment [78]. In Myanmar, patients treated by private practitioners were more likely to be LTFU [86]. An interesting situation was observed in Nigeria where patients treated at private, not-for-profit (PNFP) DOT facilities were more likely to be LTFU [87]. The researchers concluded that "Patients managed at PFP [private, for-profit] DOT facilities were probably richer, had better education, nutrition, and knowledge of TB than patients managed at PNFP

DOT facilities..." Indeed, the factors causing LTFU are not simple, and they are correlated with each other. Therefore, intervention should be addressed not only on a single problem but also targeted toward the patient as a whole. Furthermore, the provider should also be consistent throughout the different stages of treatment since different providers in the intensive phase and continuation phase are associated with LTFU [88].

5.4 Drug side effects

Studies from the USA and India have found that drug side effects are associated with LTFU [49, 77]. The researchers from the Philippines take one step further regarding this concept, stating 'patients' self-rating of the severity' as an associated factor [5]. Indeed, some side effects, such as hepatitis, of the anti-tuberculosis drugs are already severe. However, some side effects, such as vomiting, might need self-rating since different patients may perceive differently. It would be interesting to research which kind of patient rates which side effect as severe.

5.5 Social factors

Factors such as migration and social stigma also contribute toward LTFU. LTFU is common among the migrant population particularly in developed countries where there is an inward movement of people from the developing countries. Studies from the UK had repeatedly revealed this association [11, 50, 86, 89]. Researchers from the USA also found that birth outside the USA or Canada is associated with LTFU [80]. Higher LTFU among migrants has also been observed in Asian countries such as South Korea and China [70, 76, 90].

In countries where TB is a social stigma, treatment is very difficult and sensitive [77]. The patients may not want the health workers to give counseling. They do want to take treatment since the news of having TB may spread to the community, causing discrimination. In such places, secret treatment sessions should be initiated to control LTFU rates. In contrast, in Korea, the absence of TB stigma is associated with LTFU [78]. The authors wrote "TB stigma might motivate patients to receive TB treatment, thus increasing adherence to TB treatment." Therefore, before starting the TB treatment program, it is important to make community observations first to find out whether TB sigma can cause or prevent LTFU.

In theory, interpersonal factors such as family dynamics, household role, peer influence, and partner and family relationships were thought to influence LTFU [5]. However, to our knowledge, none of the studies to date supports the association of LTFU with these factors.

LTFU risk	Score
Immigration	1
Living alone	1
Living in an institution	2
Previous anti-TB treatment	2
Poor patient understanding	2
Intravenous drug use (IDU)	4
Unknown IDU status	1

Table 1.
A predictive scoring instrument for tuberculosis lost to follow-up outcome [86].

5.6 Scoring instrument

Based on the factors associated with LTFU, Rodrigo et al. have developed a scoring instrument to predict the probability of LTFU (**Table 1**) [91]. According to their original paper, "Scores of 0, 1, 2, 3, 4 and 5 points were associated with a lost to follow-up probability of 2.2% 5.4% 9.9%, 16.4%, 15%, and 28%, respectively." Incorporating the instrument in the process of history taking could help the healthcare providers in identifying patients who have the potential to be LTFU. Further interventions should be carried out to prevent these patients from becoming LTFU. Similar scoring systems could be developed in different regions, since there are always country-specific variations.

6. Interventions

6.1 Directly observed treatment (DOT)

Indeed, DOT is a part of the WHO-recommended 'Directly Observed Treatment Short Course' (DOTS) strategy. Although it cannot be denied that this strategy has saved the lives of millions of TB patients, the strategy itself is not flawless. Several authors have questioned the effectiveness of DOT as summarized in a review article by Otu [92]. The 2015 Cochrane systematic review and meta-analysis on DOT compared it with self-administered treatment, and the authors concluded that "TB cure and treatment completion were low with self-administered therapy in these trials, and direct observation did not substantially improve this" [93]. They called for complementary and alternative strategies in addition to DOT. Since DOT is a well-known and well-documented intervention in the field of TB, we felt that it need not be described in further detail in this chapter. Some interventions that have the potential to correct the weaknesses of DOT will be discussed below.

6.2 mHealth

Recently, mHealth has emerged as a popular choice for health programs around the world. The Global Observatory for eHealth (GOe) has defined mHealth as "medical and public health practice supported by mobile devices, such as mobile phones, patient monitoring devices, personal digital assistants (PDAs), and other wireless devices" [94]. Among these mHealth initiatives, appointment reminders and treatment compliance initiatives are of interest in reducing the rate of LTFU. However, there are limited interventional studies evaluating the effectiveness of these interventions in reducing the risk of LTFU.

In 2017, Hermans et al. have evaluated a text message service in the Infectious Diseases Institute (IDI) in Kampala, Uganda [95]. In this quasi-experimental study, appointment reminders were sent the day before the appointment, and adherence reminders were sent on days 2, 7, and 11 after the appointment. A total of 96% of the participants rated the messages as being helpful, and qualitative results also confirm these findings. However, data analysis has revealed that there was no statistically significant difference in the risk of LTFU between the intervention and control group. The lack of statistical significance may be due to the small sample size. Therefore, further studies with larger sample sizes are needed to further evaluate the program.

6.3 eCompliance

eCompliance is a biometric-based program, developed by Operation ASHA (OpASHA) [96], an Indian not-for-profit organization founded in 2006. The system is similar to mHealth in using text message alerts to inform the missed dose. However, the unique fingerprint verification system for the patient and the health worker takes mHealth to the next level. The OpASHA website explains the working mechanism of eCompliance as follows.

> *"During each patient visit, the patient and healthcare worker simultaneously scan their finger in the system, the medication is dispensed, and the treatment is recorded in the system's database. If a patient misses a dose, an SMS message alert is sent to the patient, healthcare worker and supervisor. The healthcare worker is then responsible to meet the patient within 24–48 hours to administer and record the treatment."*

This system can be used to reduce the risk of LTFU since the data from OpASHA stated that the LTFU rate is less than 4% using their system [96].

This claim by OpASHA has been put to test in Uganda by Snidal et al. in 2012 [97]. Community health workers (CHWs) were selected and trained to use the system. The intervention was conducted at the Millennium Villages Project (MVP) cluster in Ruhiira, Uganda. The patients were followed-up by CHWs until the end of the treatment period. The proportion of LTFU is surprisingly 0% in the intervention group, which is a significant reduction compared to the control group, yielding an excellent result. However, since this study suffers from a limited sample size, a large-scale interventional study is still necessary to confirm the results. Local adaptation to the software is available from OpASHA, and they should be incorporated into local national tuberculosis programs to lower the proportions of LTFU.

6.4 Community-based programs

An innovative community-based intervention to improve TB treatment outcomes was conducted in Sidama zone, Ethiopia [98, 99]. The core health workers mainly responsible for delivering the intervention to the grass-root level were called the health extension workers (HEWs). The HEWs were trained and salaried female health workers from the respective intervention regions. Active case finding and sputum smear preparation were conducted by the HEWs. The supervisors process the smears and initiate anti-TB treatment. Again, HEWs provide treatment support which includes provision and monitoring of treatment. Evaluation of the program over 4.5 years revealed that the proportion of patients lost to follow-up decreased significantly up to 3% [99]. The authors concluded that

> *"We have thus demonstrated that bringing simple services that detect disease and provide treatment support close to where patients live is critical to increase access to TB diagnosis and treatment adherence and minimise the number of patients LTFU."*

Therefore, such community-based programs should be implemented in modified forms in different countries around the world to reduce the proportion of LTFU. Another important thing to note is that both this program and eCompliance mentioned above employed 'task shifting' toward basic health workers (CHWs and HEWs) to support TB treatment at the grass-root level, not the experts.

6.5 Social support programs

In 2013, a novel social support program was developed in India by forming groups called "treatment support group (TSG)" [100].

> *"A TSG is a non-statutory body of socially responsible citizens and volunteers to provide social support to each needy TB patient safeguarding his dignity and confidentiality by ensuring access to information, free and quality services and social welfare programs, empowering the patient for making decision to complete the treatment successfully."*

A TSG supports the various needs of the patient so that they can complete the anti-TB treatment without any worries. The package includes transportation service, treatment counseling, emotional and spiritual support, and providing accommodation for homeless TB patients. After the program was implemented, the rate of LTFU fell until it strikes zero in the latest cohorts. It is because it tackles the social dimension associated with LTFU. This is one program that the interviewed patients from Ethiopia, who were LTFU, had hoped for [101].

6.6 Legislation

In some countries, under certain circumstances, law enforcement is controversially used to solve the problem of LTFU. Usually, the patients who were LTFU were isolated in hospitals, but in some countries, they were isolated in prisons. Usually, this method was used against patients who were homeless and had a history of alcohol abuse [102]. When all the other methods fail, the medical officer, with the power given by the health laws, has to conduct a short-term incarceration of the patients who were LTFU.

Detention of patients includes ethical and human right problems. The controversy surrounding this issue has been discussed in detail in a review article by Mburu et al. [103]. They discussed that the primary reason for detention is to protect public health, according to the Siracusa Principles adopted by the UN Economic and Social Council. However, they argued that this conflicts with the international human right laws and the 1979 Alma-Ata Declaration.

> *"...incarceration and detention approaches curtail the rights to health, informed consent, privacy, freedom from non-consensual treatment, freedom from inhumane and degrading treatment, and freedom of movement of people lost to follow-up. Detention could also worsen social inequalities and lead to a paradoxical increase in TB incidence."*

In the light of this information, the interventions which tackle the risk factors associated with LTFU are far superior to detention, which provides just a temporary solution to the problem, not a permanent one.

Another form of federal public health intervention is used in the USA to solve the problem of LTFU among the migrants [65]. These tools called the Do Not Board (DNB) and Border Lookout (BL) list are managed by the Department of Homeland Security (DHS) according to requests from the Centers for Disease Control and Prevention (CDC) Travel Restriction and Intervention expert workgroup. They are designed to detect land border travelers who were LTFU from TB treatment. State health departments and local health jurisdictions supply the list of patients and were reviewed under the following criteria:

> *"(1) infectiousness or potential infectiousness with a communicable disease that would pose a public health threat if the individual travelled internationally;*
>
> *(2) the person is unaware of his/her diagnosis, fails to adhere to public health recommendations, including treatment, or public health authorities are unable to locate the person; and*
>
> *(3) the person poses a risk to travel internationally or on a commercial flight" [65].*

Analysis revealed that most of the patients from this list were successfully treated but most of the migrants remain LTFU, suggesting that some improvement to the program is still needed to handle this problem.

7. Conclusion

LTFU from treatment is a serious problem that cannot be ignored. Throughout this chapter, the consequences of LTFU, the magnitude of this problem in different countries, and the underlying factors have been discussed. Various researchers have designed potentially powerful interventions to tackle LTFU. But, we still need further evidence and actions to be able to successfully lower the number of patients that are LTFU. With these points in mind, it is suggested that an ambitious approach should be taken to reduce the number of LTFU patients up to 0%.

Acknowledgements

I would like to thank Dr. Pa Pa Soe, associate professor, Department of Preventive and Social Medicine, University of Medicine 1, Yangon, for her invaluable advice on writing this book chapter. I am also truly grateful to Dr. Kyaw Khan Zaw, Technical Support Officer, Population Services International, Yangon, Myanmar for reviewing the chapter and giving helpful comments.

Conflict of interest

None declared.

Author details

Kyaw San Lin
University of Medicine 1, Yangon, Myanmar

*Address all correspondence to: kyawsanlin25@gmail.com

IntechOpen

© 2019 The Author(s). Licensee IntechOpen. This chapter is distributed under the terms of the Creative Commons Attribution License (http://creativecommons.org/licenses/by/3.0), which permits unrestricted use, distribution, and reproduction in any medium, provided the original work is properly cited.

References

[1] Zachariah R, Harries AD, Srinath S, Ram S, Viney K, Singogo E, et al. Language in tuberculosis services: Can we change to patient-centred terminology and stop the paradigm of blaming the patients? The International Journal of Tuberculosis and Lung Disease. 2012;**16**(6):714-717

[2] World Health Organization. Definitions and Reporting Framework for Tuberculosis–2013 Revision. 2013

[3] Baliashvili D, Magee MJ, Kempker RR, Kuchukhidze G, Aslanikashvili A, Blumberg HM. Contacts of retreatment tuberculosis cases with a prior poor treatment outcome are at increased risk of latent tuberculosis infection. International Journal of Infectious Diseases. 2016;**43**:49-50

[4] Viana PVS, Redner P, Ramos JP. Factors associated with loss to follow-up and death in cases of drug-resistant tuberculosis (DR-TB) treated at a reference center in Rio de Janeiro. Cadernos de Saúde Pública. 2018;**34**(5):e00048217

[5] Tupasi TE, Garfin AMCG, Kurbatova EV, Mangan JM, Orillaza-Chi R, Naval LC, et al. Factors associated with loss to follow-up during treatment for multidrug-resistant tuberculosis, the Philippines, 2012-2014. Emerging Infectious Diseases. 2016;**22**(3):491-502

[6] Alene KA, Yi H, Viney K, McBryde ES, Yang K, Bai L, et al. Treatment outcomes of patients with multidrug-resistant and extensively drug resistant tuberculosis in Hunan Province, China. BMC Infectious Diseases. 2017;**17**(1):573

[7] Masini EO, Mansour O, Speer CE, Addona V, Hanson CL, Sitienei JK, et al. Using survival analysis to identify risk factors for treatment interruption among new and retreatment tuberculosis patients in Kenya. PLoS One. 2016;**11**(10):e0164172

[8] Moyo S, Cox HS, Hughes J, Daniels J, Synman L, De Azevedo V, et al. Loss from treatment for drug resistant tuberculosis: Risk factors and patient outcomes in a community-based program in Khayelitsha, South Africa. PLoS One. 2015;**10**(3):e0118919. DOI: 10.1371/journal.pone.0118919

[9] Loveday M, Ramjee A, Osburn G, Master I, Kabera G, Brust JCM, et al. Drug-resistant tuberculosis in patients with minimal symptoms: Favourable outcomes in the absence of treatment. The International Journal of Tuberculosis and Lung Disease. 2017;**21**(5):556-563

[10] Trebucq A, Schwoebel V, Kashongwe Z, Bakayoko A, Kuaban C, Noeske J, et al. Treatment outcome with a short multidrug-resistant tuberculosis regimen in nine African countries. The International Journal of Tuberculosis and Lung Disease. 2018;**22**(1):17-25

[11] Millett ERC, Noel D, Mangtani P, Abubakar I, Kruijshaar ME. Factors associated with being lost to follow-up before completing tuberculosis treatment: Analysis of surveillance data. Epidemiology and Infection. 2013;**141**(6):1223-1231

[12] Randremanana RV, Richard V, Rakotomanana F, Sabatier P, Bicout DJ. Bayesian mapping of pulmonary tuberculosis in Antananarivo, Madagascar. BMC Infectious Diseases. 2010;**10**:21

[13] Dahle UR. Extensively drug resistant tuberculosis: Beware patients lost to follow-up. BMJ. 2006;**333**:705

[14] Dahle UR, Sandven P, Heldal E, Mannsaaker T, Caugant DA.

Deciphering an outbreak of drug-resistant *Mycobacterium tuberculosis*. Journal of Clinical Microbiology. 2003;**41**(1):67-72

[15] Mitruka K, Blake H, Ricks P, Miramontes R, Bamrah S, Chee C, et al. A tuberculosis outbreak fueled by cross-border travel and illicit substances: Nevada and Arizona. Public Health Reports. 2014;**129**(1):78-85

[16] Schmid D, Fretz R, Kuo H-W, Rumetshofer R, Meusburger S, Magnet E, et al. An outbreak of multidrug-resistant tuberculosis among refugees in Austria, 2005-2006. The International Journal of Tuberculosis and Lung Disease. 2008;**12**(10):1190-1195

[17] Thet Lwin ZM, Sahu SK, Owiti P, Chinnakali P, Majumdar SS. Public-private mix for tuberculosis care and control in Myanmar: A strategy to scale up? Public Health Action. 2017;7(1):15-20

[18] Gadoev J, Asadov D, Tillashaykhov M, Tayler-Smith K, Isaakidis P, Dadu A, et al. Factors associated with unfavorable treatment outcomes in new and previously treated tb patients in Uzbekistan: A five year countrywide study. PLoS One. 2015;**10**(6):e0128907

[19] Wikman-Jorgensen PE, Morales-Cartagena A, Llenas-Garcia J, Perez-Porcuna TM, Hobbins M, Ehmer J, et al. Implementation challenges of a TB programme in rural northern mozambique: Evaluation of 2012-2013 outcomes. Pathogens and Global Health. 2015;**109**(5):221-227

[20] van Lettow M, Bedell R, Maosa S, Phiri K, Chan AK, Mwinjiwa E, et al. Outcomes and diagnostic processes in outpatients with presumptive tuberculosis in Zomba District, Malawi. PLoS One. 2015;**10**(11):e0141414

[21] Wondale B, Medihn G, Teklu T, Mersha W, Tamirat M, Ameni G. A retrospective study on tuberculosis treatment outcomes at Jinka general hospital, southern Ethiopia. BMC Research Notes. 2017;**10**(1):680

[22] Conaty SJ, Dart S, Hayward AC, Lipman MC. Reasons for low reported treatment success in notified tuberculosis patients from a London hospital according to new outcome reporting. Communicable Disease and Public Health. 2004;7(1):73-76. Available from: http://www.ncbi.nlm.nih.gov/pubmed/15137286

[23] Cayla JA, Rodrigo T, Ruiz-Manzano J, Caminero JA, Vidal R, Garcia JM, et al. Tuberculosis treatment adherence and fatality in Spain. Respiratory Research. 2009;**10**:121

[24] Orenstein EW, Basu S, Shah NS, Andrews JR, Friedland GH, Moll AP, et al. Treatment outcomes among patients with multidrug-resistant tuberculosis: Systematic review and meta-analysis. The Lancet Infectious Diseases. 2009;**9**(3):153-161. DOI: 10.1016/S1473-3099(09)70041-6

[25] Johnston JC, Shahidi NC, Sadatsafavi M, Fitzgerald JM. Treatment outcomes of multidrug-resistant tuberculosis: A systematic review and meta-analysis. PLoS One. 2009;**4**(9):e6914

[26] Ahuja SD, Ashkin D, Avendano M, Banerjee R, Bauer M, Bayona JN, et al. Multidrug resistant pulmonary tuberculosis treatment regimens and patient outcomes: An individual patient data meta-analysis of 9,153 patients. PLoS Medicine. 2012;**9**(8):e1001300

[27] Anderson LF, Tamne S, Watson JP, Cohen T, Mitnick C, Brown T, et al. Treatment outcome of multi-drug resistant tuberculosis in the United Kingdom: Retrospective-prospective cohort study from 2004 to 2007. Euro Surveillance: Bulletin Europeen sur les Maladies Transmissibles = European

Communicable Disease Bulletin. 2013;**18**(40):pii=20601

[28] Jagielski T, Brzostek A, van Belkum A, Dziadek J, Augustynowicz-Kopec E, Zwolska Z. A close-up on the epidemiology and transmission of multidrug-resistant tuberculosis in Poland. European Journal of Clinical Microbiology & Infectious Diseases. 2015;**34**(1):41-53

[29] Atif M, Bashir A, Ahmad N, Fatima RK, Saba S, Scahill S. Predictors of unsuccessful interim treatment outcomes of multidrug resistant tuberculosis patients. BMC Infectious Diseases. 2017;**17**(1):655

[30] Jensenius M, Winje BA, Blomberg B, Mengshoel AT, von der Lippe B, Hannula R, et al. Multidrug-resistant tuberculosis in Norway: A nationwide study, 1995-2014. The International Journal of Tuberculosis and Lung Disease. 2016;**20**(6):786-792

[31] Cegielski JP, Kurbatova E, van der Walt M, Brand J, Ershova J, Tupasi T, et al. Multidrug-resistant tuberculosis treatment outcomes in relation to treatment and initial versus acquired second-line drug resistance. Clinical Infectious Diseases. 2016;**62**(4):418-430

[32] Gadallah MA, Mokhtar A, Rady M, El-Moghazy E, Fawzy M, Kandil SK. Prognostic factors of treatment among patients with multidrug-resistant tuberculosis in Egypt. Journal of the Formosan Medical Association. 2016;**115**(11):997-1003

[33] Kasapo CC, Chimzizi R, Simwanza SC, Mzyece J, Chizema E, Mariandyshev A, et al. What happened to patients with RMP-resistant/MDR-TB in Zambia reported as lost to follow-up from 2011 to 2014? The International Journal of Tuberculosis and Lung Disease. 2017;**21**(8):887-893

[34] Yu M-C, Chiang C-Y, Lee J-J, Chien S-T, Lin C-J, Lee S-W, et al. Treatment outcomes of multidrug-resistant tuberculosis in Taiwan: Tackling loss to follow-up. Clinical Infectious Diseases. 2018;**67**(2):202-221

[35] Huerga H, Bastard M, Kamene M, Wanjala S, Arnold A, Oucho N, et al. Outcomes from the first multidrug-resistant tuberculosis programme in Kenya. The International Journal of Tuberculosis and Lung Disease. 2017;**21**(3):314-319

[36] Alene KA, Viney K, McBryde ES, Tsegaye AT, Clements ACA. Treatment outcomes in patients with multidrug-resistant tuberculosis in north-west Ethiopia. Tropical Medicine & International Health. 2017;**22**(3):351-362

[37] Cavanaugh JS, Kazennyy BY, Nguyen ML, Kiryanova EV, Vitek E, Khorosheva TM, et al. Outcomes and follow-up of patients treated for multidrug-resistant tuberculosis in Orel, Russia, 2002-2005. The International Journal of Tuberculosis and Lung Disease. 2012;**16**(8):1069-1074

[38] Shringarpure KS, Isaakidis P, Sagili KD, Baxi RK. Loss-to-follow-up on multidrug resistant tuberculosis treatment in Gujarat, India: The when and who of it. PLoS One. 2015;**10**(7):e0132543

[39] Thu MK, Kumar AMV, Soe KT, Saw S, Thein S, Mynit Z, et al. High treatment success rate among multidrug-resistant tuberculosis patients in Myanmar, 2012-2014: A retrospective cohort study. Transactions of the Royal Society of Tropical Medicine and Hygiene. 2017;**111**(9):410-417

[40] Khaliaukin A, Kumar AMV, Skrahina A, Hurevich H, Rusovich V, Gadoev J, et al. Poor treatment outcomes among multidrug-resistant tuberculosis patients in Gomel Region, Republic of Belarus. Public Health Action. 2014;**4**(Suppl 2):S24-S28

[41] Kuchukhidze G, Kumar AMV, de Colombani P, Khogali M, Nanava U, Blumberg HM, et al. Risk factors associated with loss to follow-up among multidrug-resistant tuberculosis patients in Georgia. Public Health Action. 2014;**4**(Suppl 2):S41-S46

[42] Zhang L, Meng Q, Chen S, Zhang M, Chen B, Wu B, et al. Treatment outcomes of multidrug-resistant tuberculosis patients in Zhejiang, China, 2009-2013. Clinical Microbiology and Infection. 2018;**24**(4):381-388

[43] Parmar MM, Sachdeva KS, Dewan PK, Rade K, Nair SA, Pant R, et al. Unacceptable treatment outcomes and associated factors among India's initial cohorts of multidrug-resistant tuberculosis (MDR-TB) patients under the revised national TB control programme (2007-2011): Evidence leading to policy enhancement. PLoS One. 2018;**13**(4):e0193903

[44] Lanoix J-P, Douadi Y, Borel A, Andrejak C, El Samad Y, Ducroix J-P, et al. Lymph node tuberculosis treatment: From recommendations to practice. Médecine et Maladies Infectieuses. 2011;**41**(2):87-91

[45] Mouba JF, Miloundja J, Mimbila-Mayi M, Ndjenkam FT, N'zouba L. Cervical lymph node tuberculosis in Libreville: Epidemiology, diagnosis, and therapy. Santé. 2011;**21**(3):165-168

[46] Garg RK, Sharma R, Kar AM, Kushwaha RAS, Singh MK, Shukla R, et al. Neurological complications of miliary tuberculosis. Clinical Neurology and Neurosurgery. 2010;**112**(3):188-192

[47] AlSemari A, Baz S, Alrabiah F, Al-Khairallah T, Qadi N, Kareem A, et al. Natural course of epilepsy concomitant with CNS tuberculomas. Epilepsy Research. 2012;**99**(1-2):107-111

[48] Peluso MJ, Hung A, Lukasiewicz A, Chang H, Ramallo J, Bartlett M, et al. Successful management of latent tuberculosis infection in an underserved community by a student-run free clinic. Journal of Health Care for the Poor and Underserved. 2014 May;**25**(2):837-862

[49] Kwara A, Herold JS, Machan JT, Carter EJ. Factors associated with failure to complete isoniazid treatment for latent tuberculosis infection in Rhode Island. Chest. 2008;**133**(4):862-868

[50] Clerk N, Sisson K, Antunes G. Latent tuberculosis: Concordance and duration of treatment regimens. The British Journal of Nursing. 2011;**20**(13):824-827

[51] Langenskiold E, Herrmann FR, Luong BL, Rochat T, Janssens J-P. Contact tracing for tuberculosis and treatment for latent infection in a low incidence country. Swiss Medical Weekly. 2008;**138**(5-6):78-84

[52] Flick RJ, Kim MH, Simon K, Munthali A, Hosseinipour MC, Rosenberg NE, et al. Burden of disease and risk factors for death among children treated for tuberculosis in Malawi. The International Journal of Tuberculosis and Lung Disease. 2016;**20**(8):1046-1054

[53] Engohan Alloghe E, Toung Mve M, Ramarojoana S, Iba J, Nkoghe D. Epidemiology of childhood tuberculosis in Libreville, Gabon from 1997 to 2001. La Medicina Tropical. 2006;**66**(5):469-471

[54] Segbedji KAR, Djadou KE, Tchagbele O-B, Kpegouni M, Bessi Kama LK, Azoumah KD, et al. Tuberculosis in children in Togo: Epidemiology, diagnosis, treatment, and outcome. Medecine et Sante Tropicales. 2016;**26**(3):318-322

[55] Iroh Tam PY, Menon A, Butler K. A review of tuberculosis-related referrals among children in Ireland. Irish Journal of Medical Science. 2010;**179**(2):251-254

[56] Panigatti P, Ratageri VH, Shivanand I, Madhu PK, Shepur TA. Profile and outcome of childhood tuberculosis treated with DOTS—An observational study. Indian Journal of Pediatrics. 2014;**81**(1):9-14

[57] Pekcan S, Tana Aslan A, Kiper N, Uysal G, Gurkan F, Patiroglu T, et al. Multicentric analysis of childhood tuberculosis in Turkey. The Turkish Journal of Pediatrics. 2013;**55**(2):121-129

[58] Seddon JA, Hesseling AC, Godfrey-Faussett P, Schaaf HS. High treatment success in children treated for multidrug-resistant tuberculosis: An observational cohort study. Thorax. 2014;**69**(5):458-464

[59] Shah MA, Shah I. Increasing prevalence of pediatric drug-resistant tuberculosis in Mumbai, India and its outcome. The Pediatric Infectious Disease Journal. 2018;**37**(12):1261-1263

[60] Chiang SS, Starke JR, Miller AC, Cruz AT, Del Castillo H, Valdivia WJ, et al. Baseline predictors of treatment outcomes in children with multidrug-resistant tuberculosis: A retrospective cohort study. Clinical Infectious Diseases. 2016;**63**(8):1063-1071

[61] Horo K, Toure K, Brou-Gode V-C, Ahui BJ-M, Kouassi B-A, Gnaze A-Z, et al. Tuberculosis in the elderly: Epidemiology and outcomes of ambulatory followed-up in Abidjan. Revue d'Épidémiologie et de Santé Publique. 2012;**60**(6):484-488

[62] Laraqui CH, Ottmani S, Hammou MA, Bencheikh N, Mahjour J. Study of tuberculosis in health care workers in the public sector of Morocco. The International Journal of Tuberculosis and Lung Disease. 2001;**5**(10):939-945

[63] Adane K, Spigt M, Dinant G-J. Tuberculosis treatment outcome and predictors in northern Ethiopian prisons: A five-year retrospective analysis. BMC Pulmonary Medicine. 2018;**18**(1):37

[64] Schwitters A, Kaggwa M, Omiel P, Nagadya G, Kisa N, Dalal S. Tuberculosis incidence and treatment completion among Ugandan prison inmates. The International Journal of Tuberculosis and Lung Disease. 2014;**18**(7):781-786

[65] DeSisto C, Broussard K, Escobedo M, Borntrager D, Alvarado-Ramy F, Waterman S. Border lookout: Enhancing tuberculosis control on the United States-Mexico border. The American Journal of Tropical Medicine and Hygiene. 2015;**93**(4):747-751

[66] Gray NJ, Hansen-Knarhoi M, Krause VL. Tuberculosis in illegal foreign fishermen: Whose public health are we protecting? The Medical Journal of Australia. 2008;**188**(3):144-147

[67] Ward HA, Marciniuk DD, Hoeppner VH, Jones W. Treatment outcome of multidrug-resistant tuberculosis among Vietnamese immigrants. The International Journal of Tuberculosis and Lung Disease. 2005;**9**(2):164-169

[68] Patra S, Lukhmana S, Tayler Smith K, Kannan AT, Satyanarayana S, Enarson DA, et al. Profile and treatment outcomes of elderly patients with tuberculosis in Delhi, India: Implications for their management. Transactions of the Royal Society of Tropical Medicine and Hygiene. 2013;**107**(12):763-768

[69] Velayutham BRV, Nair D, Chandrasekaran V, Raman B, Sekar G, Watson B, et al. Profile and response to anti-tuberculosis treatment among elderly tuberculosis patients treated under the TB Control programme in South India. PLoS One. 2014;**9**(3):e88045

[70] Lin Y, Enarson DA, Du J, Dlodlo RA, Chiang C-Y, Rusen ID. Risk factors

for unfavourable treatment outcome among new smear-positive pulmonary tuberculosis cases in China. Public Health Action. 2017;**7**(4):299-303

[71] Enane LA, Lowenthal ED, Arscott-Mills T, Matlhare M, Smallcomb LS, Kgwaadira B, et al. Loss to follow-up among adolescents with tuberculosis in Gaborone, Botswana. The International Journal of Tuberculosis and Lung Disease. 2016;**20**(10):1320-1325

[72] Dangisso MH, Datiko DG, Lindtjorn B. Trends of tuberculosis case notification and treatment outcomes in the Sidama Zone, southern Ethiopia: Ten-year retrospective trend analysis in urban-rural settings. PLoS One. 2014;**9**(12):e114225

[73] Javaid A, Shaheen Z, Shafqat M, Khan AH, Ahmad N. Risk factors for high death and loss-to-follow-up rates among patients with multidrug-resistant tuberculosis at a programmatic management unit. American Journal of Infection Control. 2017;**45**(2):190-193

[74] Bemba ELP, Bopaka RG, Ossibi-Ibara R, Toungou SN, Ossale-Abacka BK, Okemba-Okombi FH, et al. Predictive factors of lost to follow-up status during tuberculosis treatment in Brazzaville. Revue de Pneumologie Clinique. 2017;**73**(2):81-89

[75] Mainbourg EMT, Belchior ADS, Goncalves MJF. Loss to follow-up in tuberculosis treatment and its relationship with patients' knowledge of the disease and other associated factors. Rev Salud Pública. 2017;**18**(5):714. Available from: http://www.ncbi.nlm.nih.gov/pubmed/28453113

[76] Li T, Zhang H, Wang LX, Pang Y, DU X. Description and factors affecting the referral of presumptive tuberculosis patients in China. Biomedical and Environmental Sciences. 2017;**30**(6):444-449

[77] Deshmukh RD, Dhande DJ, Sachdeva KS, Sreenivas A, Kumar AMV, Satyanarayana S, et al. Patient and provider reported reasons for lost to follow up in MDRTB treatment: A qualitative study from a drug resistant TB centre in India. PLoS One. 2015;**10**(8):e0135802

[78] Park C-K, Shin H-J, Kim Y-I, Lim S-C, Yoon J-S, Kim Y-S, et al. Predictors of default from treatment for tuberculosis: A single center case-control study in Korea. Journal of Korean Medical Science. 2016;**31**(2):254-260

[79] Brainard D, Hyslop NE, Mera R, Churchill J. Long-term outcome of inpatients with tuberculosis assigned to outpatient therapy at a local clinic in New Orleans. Journal of Investigative Medicine. 1997;**45**(6):381-387

[80] Conwell DS, Mosher A, Khan A, Tapy J, Sandman L, Vernon A, et al. Factors associated with loss to follow-up in a large tuberculosis treatment trial (TBTC Study 22). Contemporary Clinical Trials. 2007;**28**(3):288-294

[81] Story A, Murad S, Roberts W, Verheyen M, Hayward AC. Tuberculosis in London: The importance of homelessness, problem drug use and prison. Thorax. 2007;**62**(8):667-671

[82] Ogbudebe CL, Izuogu S, Abu CE. Magnitude and treatment outcomes of pulmonary tuberculosis patients in a poor urban slum of Abia State, Nigeria. International Journal of Mycobacteriology. 2016;**5**(2):205-210

[83] Ade S, Harries AD, Trebucq A, Ade G, Agodokpessi G, Adjonou C, et al. National profile and treatment outcomes of patients with extrapulmonary tuberculosis in Benin. PLoS One. 2014;**9**(4):e95603

[84] Mi F, Tan S, Liang L, Harries AD, Hinderaker SG, Lin Y, et al. Diabetes

mellitus and tuberculosis: Pattern of tuberculosis, two-month smear conversion and treatment outcomes in Guangzhou, China. Tropical Medicine & International Health. 2013;**18**(11):1379-1385

[85] Asres A, Jerene D, Deressa W. Delays to treatment initiation is associated with tuberculosis treatment outcomes among patients on directly observed treatment short course in Southwest Ethiopia: A follow-up study. BMC Pulmonary Medicine. 2018;**18**(1):64

[86] Nwe TT, Saw S, Le Win L, Mon MM, van Griensven J, Zhou S, et al. Engagement of public and private medical facilities in tuberculosis care in Myanmar: Contributions and trends over an eight-year period. Infectious Diseases of Poverty. 2017;**6**(1):123

[87] Adejumo OA, Daniel OJ, Otesanya AF, Salisu-Olatunj SO, Abdur-Razzaq HA. Evaluation of outcomes of tuberculosis management in private for profit and private-not-for profit directly observed treatment short course facilities in Lagos State, Nigeria. Nigerian Medical Journal. 2017;**58**(1):44-49

[88] Shringarpure KS, Isaakidis P, Sagili KD, Baxi RK. Loss-to-follow-up on multidrug resistant tuberculosis treatment in Gujarat, India: The when and who of it. PLoS One. 2015;**10**(7):1-10

[89] Anyama N, Bracebridge S, Black C, Niggebrugge A, Griffin SJ. What happens to people diagnosed with tuberculosis? A population-based cohort. Epidemiology and Infection. 2007;**135**(7):1069-1076

[90] Min GH, Kim Y, Lee JS, Oh JY, Hur GY, Lee YS, et al. Social and clinical characteristics of immigrants with tuberculosis in South Korea. Yonsei Medical Journal. 2017;**58**(3):592-597

[91] Rodrigo T, Cayla JA, Casals M, Garcia-Garcia JM, Caminero JA, Ruiz-Manzano J, et al. A predictive scoring instrument for tuberculosis lost to follow-up outcome. Respiratory Research. 2012;**13**:75

[92] Asuquo Otu A. Is the directly observed therapy short course (DOTS) an effective strategy for tuberculosis control in a developing country? Asian Pacific Journal of Tropical Medicine. 2013;**3**(3):227-231

[93] Karumbi J, Garner P. Directly observed therapy for treating tuberculosis. Cochrane Database of Systematic Reviews. 2015;**5**:CD003343

[94] World Health Organization. mHealth: New Horizons for Health Through Mobile Technologies. World Health Organization; 2011

[95] Hermans SM, Elbireer S, Tibakabikoba H, Hoefman BJ, Manabe YC. Text messaging to decrease tuberculosis treatment attrition in TB-HIV coinfection in Uganda. Patient Preference and Adherence. 2017;**11**:1479-1487

[96] Operation ASHA. eCOMPLIANCE [Internet]. 2018. Available from: https://www.opasha.org/blog/2016/09/20/ecompliance-biometric-tracking-system/ [Accessed: 01 September 2018]

[97] Snidal SJ, Barnard G, Atuhairwe E, Ben AY. Use of eCompliance, an innovative biometric system for monitoring of tuberculosis treatment in rural Uganda. The American Journal of Tropical Medicine and Hygiene. 2015;**92**(6):1271-1279

[98] Yassin MA, Datiko DG, Tulloch O, Markos P, Aschalew M, Shargie EB, et al. Innovative community-based approaches doubled tuberculosis case notification and improve treatment outcome in southern Ethiopia. PLoS One. 2013;**8**(5):1-8

[99] Datiko DG, Yassin MA, Theobald SJ, Blok L, Suvanand S, Creswell J, et al. Health extension workers improve tuberculosis case finding and treatment outcome in Ethiopia: A large-scale implementation study. BMJ Global Health. 2017;**2**(4):e000390

[100] Balakrishnan S, Manikantan J, Sreenivas A, Jayasankar S, Sunilkumar M, Rakesh PS, et al. Social inclusion: An effort to end loss-to-treatment follow-up in tuberculosis. The Indian Journal of Tuberculosis. 2015;**62**(4):230-234

[101] Getahun B, Nkosi ZZ. Is directly observed tuberculosis treatment strategy patient-centered? a mixed method study in Addis Ababa, Ethiopia. PLoS One. 2017;**12**(8):e0181205

[102] Burman WJ, Cohn DL, Rietmeijer CA, Judson FN, Sbarbaro JA, Reves RR. Short-term incarceration for the management of noncompliance with tuberculosis treatment. Chest. 1997;**112**(1):57-62

[103] Mburu G, Restoy E, Kibuchi E, Holland P, Harries AD. Detention of people lost to follow-up on tb treatment in Kenya: The need for human rights-based alternatives. Health and Human Rights. 2016;**18**(1):43-54

Chapter 9

An Update on Cholera Studies in Mozambique

Edgar Manuel Cambaza, Edson Mongo, Elda Anapakala, Robina Nhambire, Jacinto Singo and Edsone Machava

Abstract

Cholera is endemic in Mozambique and, together with other diarrheic diseases, is a major cause of infant death. There are yearly outbreaks in the northern provinces. The last major review of cholera in the country was published in 2013, but there have been major events since then, such as the 2015 outbreak in central and northern Mozambique and others in the following years. Plenty of related information were shared during the XVI National Health Journeys, 17–20 September 2018, in Maputo City. This chapter aims to summarize and discuss the most relevant information on cholera from the journeys, and other recent publications, in order to update the information from the latest major review. Regarding etiology, new strains of *V. cholerae* irradiating from several areas have been replacing the original from the Indian subcontinent. Water and sanitation are major challenges but, in some instances, sociocultural features play a significant role in people's reluctance to use untreated water, even when they have access to potable sources, and mistrust toward government interventions. Vaccination campaigns seemed effective but there is a need to promote more adherence and collaboration from people at risk, perhaps by involving more the local government and religious and traditional authorities.

Keywords: cholera, diarrhea, Mozambique, update, epidemiology

1. Introduction

Diarrheic diseases are a serious public health issue in the entire world [1, 2]. Cholera is among the deadliest gastrointestinal diarrheic maladies in tropical areas [3–5], resulting almost exclusively from ingestion of water contaminated with *Vibrio cholerae*, but any fecal-oral pathway can potentially transmit the disease [6]. When untreated, the disease rapidly results in death, and transmission is quick within the community [2]. It is a problem because many developing countries lack resources and time necessary for confirmation and management of cholera outbreaks [7].

In the African continent, cholera has been a significant cause of morbidity and mortality [3, 6]. The disease was introduced in Mozambique from the Indian subcontinent in 1970 and became a major cause of infectious diarrhea [4, 8, 9]. Since then, the country has been facing outbreaks, particularly in Nampula Province [6]. The most severe happened during the 1990s, resulting in one third of all cases in Africa [5]. All diarrheic diseases together are the fourth major cause of death of <5-year-old children, causing in average 13,105 demises per annum. Cholera's epidemiological profile is changed from epidemic to endemic due to the frequent outbreaks [6]. In general, there is a virtually countrywide epidemics every 5 years, but Nampula and Cuamba cities register annual cases [1], usually during the rainy season (December to June) [8]. According to Chissaque et al. [10], the last major outbreak was in 2015. Furthermore, some issues have been worsening the situation and raising increased concern. For instance, diarrhea-causing enteric bacteria are developing resistance to antibiotics [11], possibly because of overprescription.

Cholera is endemic in Mozambique, but there is very limited research on the matter. There is little information on transmission patterns and how risk factors such as non-potable water, improper sanitation, and hygiene affect the incidence, prevalence, and severity of the disease [4, 9]; there is no local protocol for treating acute diarrhea in children, the only reference being from the World Health Organization (WHO) [4, 12, 13]; little is known about the challenges, success cases, and the extent of the impact of the struggle against cholera in Mozambique [2] and the operational cost to implement a vaccination campaign against cholera [14]. If such information gaps are filled, it will be possible to substantially improve the strategy to mitigate the disease.

Gujral et al. [15] wrote an important contribution to the overall understanding of cholera epidemiology in Mozambique up to 2013, based on the national surveillance data. Though it is a good reference for researchers and scholars, there were some updates published in at least three journal articles [9, 10, 16], reports from the United Nations [17] or other organizations, and 17 presentations [1–8, 11, 14, 18–24] at the XVI Scientific Journeys organized by the Mozambican National Institute of Health [25]. This chapter aims to summarize the contributions of such publications for the current knowledge of cholera in Mozambique.

2. Sources and reviewing process

The current analysis is based on updates presented during the XVI National Health Journeys, 17–20 September 2018, in Maputo City, in Mozambique. National Health Institute organized the event under the motto "Promovendo a intersectorialidade e a participação comunitária para o alcance dos Objectivos de Desenvolvimento Sustentável" [Promoting the multi-sectoral collaboration and community participation to meet the Sustainable Development Goals]. Since the beginning, in 1976, the journeys have been arguably the country's most relevant event on the matter, hosting presentations from leading health researchers in Mozambique [26].

Summaries of all presentations were then compiled to Revista Moçambicana de Ciências de Saúde [Mozambican Journal of Health Sciences]. There were 19 presentations directly or indirectly related to cholera. Some content was a follow-up of other previously published international journals, and it facilitated their interpretation. ATLAS.ti 8.1 (ATLAS.ti Scientific Software Development GmbH, Berlin, Germany) was used to analyze most information and Jamovi 0.9 (The Jamovi Project, Amsterdam, Netherlands) for meta-analysis when necessary.

Most studies on cholera in Mozambique conducted during the last decade were complementary, connected as part of a multidisciplinary approach for accompanying control campaigns led by the Ministry of Health, targeted to susceptible groups in areas where annual outbreaks occur during the rainy season [16]. At least half of the studies used data from Nampula City [23], but there were also studies in Tete, Moatize, Quelimane, Mocuba, Guruè, Metangula, Cuamba, and the country in general [1, 2, 5, 19–21]. Chissaque and Deus [20] presented, in the journeys, content directly related to a journal article published the same year [10].

It is perhaps important to mention the group that contributed the most with presentations about cholera during the Scientific Journeys. It was the team of Baltazar and Baloi [23], from the National Institute of Health, mostly reporting on different aspects of the immunization campaign in Nampula City, 2016. Their particular presentation was focused on the vaccine coverage and acceptability, but the same group also analyzed local media coverage and people's reaction [21], evaluated environmental determinants [4] and post-campaign adverse effects [18], validated a rapid test to monitor the efficacy of the vaccine [7], and evaluated the economic cost of the vaccine [14].

3. The current situation of cholera in Mozambique

Since most publications are interconnected, based on the same campaigns and projects, they shared some constraints and limitations. They might not be explored in full depth in the following subsections. Section 5.7.3 presents more details and respective analyses on the limitations and constraints.

3.1 Etiology

The main causes of diarrhea in Mozambique, especially in children, are *V. cholerae,* rotavirus, *Shigella* spp., *Escherichia coli*, *Cryptosporidium* spp., and *Aeromonas* spp. [20]. At this stage, *V. cholerae* is well-known as the cholera-causing microorganism, even outside scholarly or scientific circles. Etiological studies are now focused on peculiarities or diversity of endemic strains in Mozambique, and how to rapidly distinguish cases of cholera from other forms of diarrhea, especially during emergency situations. The more accurate the diagnostic, the more appropriate the treatment.

According to Langa et al. [16], Mozambican *V. cholerae* O1 isolates from 2012 to 2014 outbreaks are genetically closely related to strains of pandemic worldwide, unlike the Indian-born found 20 years ago. Garrine et al. [9] went one step forward by analyzing how related 75 isolated were from patients in Manhiça District Hospital from the start of the millennium up to 2012 and 3 from the Komati River. They were able to reveal four unrelated genotypes and two clonal complexes with 22 genotypes by using a multilocus variable-number tandem-repeat analysis (MLVA), and through whole genome sequencing (WGS), they detected recombination and four isolates genetically unable to produce cholera toxin. The investigators were also able to deduct that Wave 3 of the seventh pandemic [27–29] remained in the area for at least 8 years, originating 67 of the isolates analyzed.

It is worth mentioning *Aeromonas* spp., as Chitio and Langa [24] demonstrated that these microorganisms cause symptoms easy to confuse with cholera's, particularly during outbreaks. They detected *Aeromonas* spp. in 30 (10.4%) of 289 samples of rectal swabs from patients with suspicion of cholera during outbreaks in 2014 and 2015. The species were *Aeromonas sobria* (57%), *Aeromonas hydrophila* (20%), *Aeromonas caviae* (13%), *Aeromonas veronii* (7%), and *Aeromonas salmonicida* ssp. *salmonicida* (3%).

3.2 Risk factors and health determinants

Environmental sanitation is important to control disease for the benefit of public health [19]. For several natural, sociopolitical, cultural, and economic reasons, Mozambique is spatially heterogeneous in terms of distribution of resources, including water, housing, their conditions [30], and certainly other features potentially affecting the transmission of cholera. Thus, one shall expect to see substantial differences in terms of risk factors and health determinants in different areas throughout the country. Yet, it is possible to draw some comparisons on how one or another factor affects the dynamics of cholera transmissibility, from different authors' points of view.

Marrufo et al. [4] evaluated water, sanitation, and hygiene in the area with more cases of cholera in Nampula City and found that 42% had improved latrines and 90% of the inhabitants had access to at least one improved water source, as defined by the World Health Organization and the United Nations Children's Fund (UNICEF) [31]: with potential to deliver safe water by nature of its design and construction. The authors did not specify their sample size (n) in the summary for the presentation, but their sample was certainly representative because they followed the guidelines of the United Nations High Commissioner for Refugees, and they were the same research team as Baltazar et al. [23] (n = 636), besides the fact that they covered a very wide area and used a statistical treatment of the data. A major health determinant is likely the lack of drainage and sewage through the entire suburban area covering six neighborhoods, particularly when it rains [4, 8, 20]. According to Ramos et al. [19], residents of Bairro Novo [New Neighborhood], Quelimane City, claimed to frequently observe human stool and trash floating when it rains and water accumulates through the streets. This area also lacks a sewage system and has a shortage of latrines.

A different research team [22] interviewed 59 patients with suspicion of cholera in the rural community of Casacone and found the same percentage as Marrufo et al. [4] of households with latrines (42%), but there were differences: 64% used well water, and none treated it before consuming. Besides the differences in the settings (suburban and rural), the study groups were fundamentally different, as Paulo et al. [22] worked with people having acute diarrhea, while Marrufo et al. [4] worked with populations from a risky area. The former group was by definition people who had contact with contaminated water; thus it is not surprising that all used untreated water, unlike the latter group.

Borges et al. [5] found that people in Metangula District (Niassa Province) prefer using untreated water from the lake, even when they have access to potable water, and they could not find any explanation, particularly because most (98%) were aware of cholera and the associated risks. Adding to that fact, Francisco and Chindia [3] stated that in this particular area, temperature and precipitation do not seem to be major health determinants, and it reinforces the idea that the issue is led by behavior. There are perhaps sociocultural or religious reasons. For instance, the Zion Christian Church is well-known in Mozambique, and it is the third largest (17.5% of the population), only surpassed by Catholicism (23.8%) and Islam (17.8%) [32]. One notable ritual of this church is the "Jordan" baptism, performed in rivers, lakes, and sometimes the sea. Such level of exposition to waterborne pathogens is highly concerning, particularly in hotspots of cholera endemism. Furthermore, virtually all over Mozambique, there are people who believe that malicious individuals intentionally created cholera to harm others [2, 6, 33]. Thus, it is important to debunk such self-destructive mentality and the resulting attitudes.

3.3 Epidemiology

3.3.1 Geographical distribution

The World Health Organization [34] identifies Mozambique among the African countries most affected by cholera epidemics. In the first decade of the millennium, cholera had an incidence of 12 to 127 per 100,000 inhabitants, especially in the rainy season [20]. The variant of *V. cholerae* O1 (El Tor strains) active in the country then came from the Indian subcontinent, and it can be found, for instance, in Bangladesh

[16, 35]. Between 25 December 2014 and 22 March 2015, there was a sequence of outbreaks through 5 provinces and 18 districts, resulting in 7073 cases reported and 53 deaths (fatality rate was 0.7%) [17]. Genetic analyses suggest that strains found in Mozambique since 2012 are also common in several other parts of the world [16], indicating the existence of different waves of contamination converging in the country.

Chitio and Langa [24] and several other presenters in the XVI National Health Journeys seemed to agree that cholera has been more widespread throughout the central and northern provinces (**Figure 1**), particularly Niassa and Nampula in the north, where outbreaks occur annually, in contrast to the rest of the country, where it occurs every 5 years [1, 4, 22].

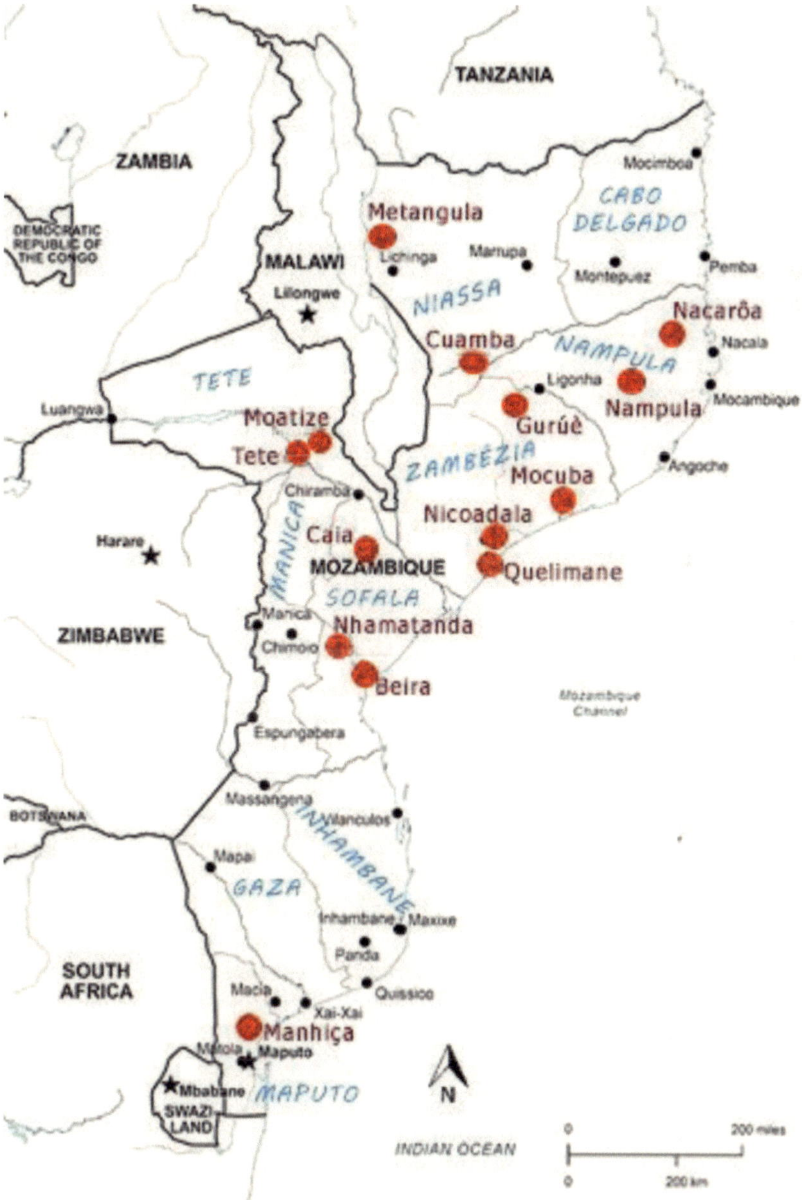

Figure 1.
Draft of Mozambican map showing the areas where research and interventions related to cholera occurred since 2013. Image adapted from Wikimedia Commons [36] under public domain. Data was compiled from the XVI National Health Journeys [1–8, 11, 14, 18–24], Chissaque et al. [10], and Vanormelingen et al. [17].

Vanormelingen et al. [17] included Sofala in the list of affected provinces, and Chissaque et al. [20] mentioned *V. cholerae* among the causes of diarrhea in the country's south. The main cause is the lack of potable water and proper sanitation such as improved latrines [4], though behavioral factors also contribute to the incidence and prevalence of cholera [6, 8, 21].

In Niassa Province, the most frequent reports have arisen from in two municipalities: Metangula, where the majority of the cases occur [5], and Cuamba [1]. Besides similar causes as in Nampula City, a major risk factor for cholera contamination in Niassa is the insistence on using untreated fresh water to wash dishes, take a bath, and drink, especially the population of Metangula who live at the Niassa lakeshore [5]. In their presentation, Borges et al. [5] stated that choice of fresh water is not necessarily related to the access to potable water, as there were sufficient wells for the community.

In Nampula, the six most severely affected neighborhood cities are Carrupeia, Muatala, Murrapaniua, Mutauanha, Napipine, and Natiquiri, with 193.403 inhabitants [1, 4, 18]. Other neighborhoods under risk are Namicopo, Namutequeliua, and Belenenses, especially considering a recent observation that some residents showed very low awareness on how cholera is transmitted [6]. In this decade, the city had annual outbreaks recorded at least from 2013 to 2018 [4], and it is confirmed that an outbreak is happening as this article is being written [37], but this topic will be briefly discussed in the post-conclusion note (Section 7). There was another outbreak notified 17 November 2017 in Nampula Province, Nacarôa District [22]. The most affected areas were Munana and Casaconde neighborhoods, in the administrative area also called Nacarôa, within the district.

Zambezia was another province studied, and there were studies from cities of Quelimane, Mocuba, and Gurúè [1, 2, 19]. Vanormelingen et al. [17] added Nicoadala District. First, regarding "Bairro Novo" [New Neighborhood] in Quelimane City, Ramos et al. [19] mentioned the rapid expansion of the city, hardly complying with proper urbanization planning, thus resulting in improper sanitation and hygiene. The authors decided to investigate the frequency of waterborne diseases, including diarrheic maladies, by interviewing members of 21 households, and analyzing records from the Healthcare Center from 24 July 2014 to 2017. Cholera was mentioned among the most frequent diseases, although the authors did not specify the prevalence. In general, they included the disease among the diarrheic, with 564 cases (47.3%) in 1193 recorded in the healthcare center's registry. In Mocuba, Mesa et al. [1] analyzed 128 processes of patients carrying diarrheic diseases. Although the authors did not specify the diseases, they suspected that most had cholera considering the symptoms recorded, the fatality rate of 4% (plausible, according to the World Health Organization [38]), and the fact that there was an outbreak as they were conducting their investigation. The most affected neighborhoods were Samora Machel (33%), Marmanelo (15%), CFM (11%), carreira de tiros (10%), and Tomba de Água (8%). Carlos [2] said that various minor towns of Gurúè District have been registering outbreaks of diarrheic diseases and cholera, but in 2015 there was an outbreak in its main city, also called Gurúè.

There are other areas where cholera is endemic, but the scholarly publications from the last decade did not explore in depth the epidemiologic point of view, but they are worth mentioning. For instance, the 2015 outbreaks in the country's north and center seemed interconnected and occurred during the same period, and they reached areas including the cities of Tete, Moatize, and Sofala Province [17]. There are also studies from the south, though in different time and context. Salomão et al. [21] presented results of a 2-year study (2017–2018) related to immunization campaigns in the cities of Tete and Moatize, after an outbreak in 2017. As the outbreaks were stabilizing in the provinces mentioned so far, in Sofala it was spreading, with reports from Beira City, Caia, and Nhamatanda. Manhiça District Hospital keeps isolates of cholera [9], and it reflects the history of the disease there and in the areas nearby. Garrine et al. [9] worked with these isolates in their research and added three from the Komati River.

3.3.2 Prevalence, impact, and susceptible groups

Since most studies presented at the XVI Health Journeys were follow-ups of ongoing studies, they all tended to miss some details, and some were complementary to each other. For instance, the studies after the 2015 outbreak of cholera in Nampula explored different perspectives on the problematics [4, 6–8, 14, 18, 22, 23]. **Table 1** shows some epidemiological data recorded after 2013. These are just some examples because it would be redundant to include some papers, particularly the studies conducted in Nampula. Still, there is plenty of information worth sharing.

The studies did not explain the dynamics of how the disease is spread during non-epidemic periods because virtually all were conducted during outbreaks, or at least based on them, though it might not differ much from times of outbreak, especially because the area is endemic. Phenomena such as heavy rain and natural catastrophes certainly work as amplifiers of the disease severity by increasing people's exposition to untreated water [3, 20, 39–42]. Yet, it would be a good idea to study the risk factors and disease determinants during times of low prevalence because it would, for instance, minimize the need for researchers to work under pressure or "under budget" because of non-research-driven priorities [43], avoid panic or undesirable reactions from study subjects, and perhaps be easy to prevent outbreaks or lower considerably their impact on public health. On the other hand, outbreak investigations are crucial to ensure proper intervention. Thus, the information below represents outbreak-related scenarios but somehow the best lead so far of the country's reality with or without an outbreak.

According to **Table 1**, the country's cholera fatality rate (CFR) in 2015 was 0.7%. This value is low, within the range 0–15.8% of the Global Health Observatory (GHO) in 2016, published by the World Health Organization [38]. According to the GHO, 22 countries had CFR > 1%, and only Niger, Zimbabwe, and Congo had CFR > 5%. Even the global (1.8%) was higher than Mozambique the previous year during the outbreak. Such low fatality rate was likely due to a very fast and effective response in terms of vaccination, treatment [11, 23], and other measures such as health education and support in sanitation [8, 17]. Cholera is highly virulent but also easy to treat and there is vaccine [44]. The fatality rate observed in Nacarôa (2%) was not far from the global, and it seems reasonable to expect such kind of fluctuations in a considerably small sample. It should be also reasonable to expect a value slightly higher than average in endemic areas.

Author	Year	Area	Cases of cholera	Deaths
Vanormelingen et al. [17]	2015	Countrywide	7073	53
Salência et al. [11]	2014–2017	Countrywide (6 hospitals)	19/784*	ns
Dengo-Baloi et al. [18]	2016	Nampula City	44/171*	ns
Paulo et al. [22]	2017	Nacarôa	135	3

**Confirmed cases/suspected cases in children recorded in healthcare institutions; ns, non-specified.*

Table 1.
Cases of cholera recorded in the decade so far.

It is general knowledge that cholera is spread through water and improper sanitation is a major risk factor for transmission. Thus, the disease deeply related to poverty in several ways including obviously the lack of resources for prevention or treatment and limitations in education or information. It is intuitive that the most susceptible are people living in highly crowded suburban areas when people have little access to clean water, or in rural settings, when people directly consume water from lakes or rivers without any treatment. People living around Lake Niassa use it for domestic purposes [5]. This is the reality in several areas of Mozambique. This must be understood on top of any specificity of the studies explained or discussed in this subsection. It must be implicit that all the studies' target populations were susceptible to cholera.

The research team of Baltazar et al. [23] belongs to the National Institute of Health, and they conducted most studies related to the vaccination campaign in Nampula City, 2016. In the particular study cited, they focused on inhabitants over 1 year old living in the city's six most susceptible neighborhoods, mentioned in Section 5.4.1 (Geographical distribution). People from surrounding areas are also at risk [4] because of mobility and interaction with residents of the endemic neighborhoods or exchange of food or drinks coming from such zones.

Children are the most susceptible to diarrheic diseases in general [11, 20] perhaps because of their immunity still under development, their unawareness of the bacterial load in the untreated water, and their behavior. In reality, they have always been the priority and focus of the vaccination campaigns [10, 45]. Among 1910 children hospitalized with acute diarrhea from May 2014 to December 2017, Salência et al. [11] found that <1-year-olds were the most affected and 19 infants (2.4%) had *V. cholerae*. The majority (58%) were male, but it seems that the proportion male/female always gravitates around 1:1 [1, 11, 22]. Mesa et al. [1] analyzed 128 processes of patients with acute diarrhea in Mocuba District Hospital, admitted during June and July 2015 in the local hospital. According to the authors, all patients presented symptoms consistent with cholera, but, despite their convictions, there was no confirmation, and they based their conclusions on clinical data (aqueous stool, vomit, and fever). In any case, all were below 16 years old in which 41% were below 5 years and 4% of the cases ended in decease. Differently, Paulo et al. [22] found 68% of individuals over 15 years old among 135 cases of cholera in the Center for Treatment of Diarrheic Diseases in Nacarôa District, recorded from 12 to 28 November 2017. The difference is likely due to a fact mentioned by the authors that none treated the water before consuming and the majority (64%) used well water. One has to imagine that the entire household uses the same water source and all the members have nearly the same level of exposition if it is contaminated, independently of the age and behavior of each individual. The age or sex differences might be a reflection of the actual sociodemographic profile of the community.

3.4 Diagnosis

There is little novelty on diagnosis in Mozambique since the beginning of the decade. It is perhaps worth mentioning that during the 2016 massive vaccination campaign in Nampula, Dengo-Baloi et al. [18] performed a rapid test to verify if it could be an alternative to the culture-based standard, as the latter takes 48 to 72 hours and the rapid test would take approximately 6 hours. They used an alkaline peptone water (APW) enrichment method, but they did not specify the origin of the kit. It was likely Crystal VC RDT (Span Divergent, Mumbai, India), previously used by George et al. [46] in Bangladesh and Ontweka et al. [47] in South Sudan. According to the latter, it is also considerably inexpensive. Dengo-Baloi et al. [18]

observed exactly the same results using the standard method and the rapid test for 75 samples, demonstrating its efficacy as a good alternative for the standard in areas with limited resources.

3.5 Control strategies

3.5.1 Overview, prophylaxis, and awareness

Cholera control strategies in Mozambique have been changing over time, perhaps due to governmental priorities, an increasing knowledge, or resources available. Regarding Mozambique, it is important to keep in mind that Mozambique has undergone major political changes, there have been conflicts, including armed, natural calamities such as drought, floods, typhoons, economic crises, and fluctuations. All these phenomena resulted in mobility or affected people's livelihoods, changing the dynamics of access to resources, including potable water, ultimately impacting public health. This ever-changing environment has been determining, at a certain extent, the way the government deals with the epidemics of infectious diseases, including cholera. Chissaque et al. [20] mentioned some key actions of the government's strategy: vaccination, health education, introduction of zinc and salts for oral hydration, improvement of basic sanitation (construction of latrines and access to potable water), and organization of national health weeks. Dengo-Baloi et al. [18] added vigilance among the measures, and Vanormelingen et al. [17] said that the government coordinated a real-time mapping of the epidemic and supported social mobilization with the assistance of the United Nations Children's Fund, World Health Organization, and Médecins Sans Frontières (MSF).

The most relevant actions in the last decade are perhaps related to the Ministry of Health's implementation of vaccination campaigns using Shanchol™ (BivWC, Shantha [48], Ranga Reddy District, Telangana, India) in Nampula City's six most vulnerable neighborhoods, in October 2016 and also the subsequent years [4, 10, 21]. It was in response to the outbreak in 2015, and the strategy was to deliver the vaccine door to door in two rounds [23]. Paulo et al. [22] mentioned another outbreak in November 2017, but it did not seem as severe. The 2016 campaign was strategically set to cover 193,403 individuals and prevent the expansion of cholera to less affected areas [4, 18]. Though the first round only covered 69.5% of the target population, and the second covered 51.2%, Baltazar et al. [23] considered the experience as a success and shared the belief that similar strategies can have more adherence in urban settings when there is no emergency. Considerably low adherence was mostly because many people were not at home during the campaign, and 17.3% of 636 people enquired said that they were unaware of the campaign. The situation was similar in the following 2 years [21]. Thus, it is important to improve or use more effectively the channels to communicate with the residents.

After vaccination, there were adverse effects such as abdominal pain, nausea, and diarrhea, but none seemed severe enough to require any medical assistance [18]. The National Institute of Health organized a vigilance of postimmunization adverse effects in nine healthcare units, and, according to Dengo-Baloi et al. [18], there were eight cases reported after the first round of vaccination, three during the second, and one case during both rounds. Yet, there were certainly more cases because Baltazar et al. [23] reported adverse effects in 47 people of 451 interviewed after receiving vaccination. A possible explanation for the discrepancy between both studies is the fact that PIAE vigilance recorded mostly cases that occurred 24 h after vaccination, and it was based on records from healthcare units, while the other study was based on inquiries directly to randomly chosen individuals from the community from 2 to 9 November 2016 [18, 23].

Among the 428 interviewees of Borges et al. [5] in Metangula, the level of awareness on cholera was very high (98%), and they said that radio (35%) and lectures at the healthcare center (28%) were the main sources of information about the disease. If the population in general is aware of the disease and still Metangula is the town most affected with cholera in Niassa Province, perhaps most inhabitants lack essential knowledge on how to prevent the disease or have very few alternatives as source of water or means to properly treat it. Yet, the investigators claim that most people from Metangula have access to potable water, but they prefer the untreated from the Lake Niassa and proposed further studies to understand their motivation. They also believe that it is necessary to intensify awareness campaigns on how to prevent cholera. However, such campaigns might not be very effective if people mistrust the authorities, as Victorino et al. [6] said. The latter authors interviewed 30 residents throughout three neighborhoods of Nampula City (the same region of the country), and they unanimously claimed that the government was responsible for the outbreak of cholera. Furthermore, the majority (18 people) did not really understand the concept of cholera (bacterial disease transmitted through water), and 12 did not know how to prevent the disease. In this case, it would be more prudent to approach the residents through authorities they might be more prone to trust, such as teachers at schools, traditional leaders and religious entities.

3.5.2 Constraints and limitations

At a first glance, the main constraints seem related to vaccination, improper treatment and potential misdiagnosis of diarrheic diseases, unclear notion on the impact of risk factors, shortage of resources for interventions, and government mistrust. Some constraints might be related, and for this reason they will not be necessarily presented in the same order as mentioned. This subsection might seem redundant in the sense that it recapitulates some limitations from the previous subsections. However, it seems important to discuss them in more detail, as they are likely to be the starting point for future researchers aiming to study the dynamics of cholera epidemiology and control strategies in Mozambique. Furthermore, some ideas are consolidated, and some relationships are explored more critically in this subsection.

According to Baltazar et al. [23], during the 2016 vaccination campaign in Nampula, more than one third missed the vaccine because they were not at home or did not receive any information prior to the campaign, and in the second round, there were less people available, though dropout rates from the first to the second dose up to 13% is not uncommon due to factors such as migration or other reasons leading people to be absent [49, 50]. Salomão et al. [21] stated that it happened again the following year, and, according to them, the main reasons were lack of time, absence, and lack of information. The overall vaccine wastage rate was 10%, and it seems high if compared with the experience in Bangladesh between February and April 2011, where it was 1.2% [49]. Such wastage might be partially related to reasons to be discussed in the following paragraph.

It seems important to discuss the most likely motivation for the vaccination campaign's suboptimal adherence. Since the strategy was door to door, it seems difficult to suddenly receive someone claiming to be from the government and offering substances to all family members including children. Even if the visitors show credentials, many inhabitants mistrust the government and blame it for the disease [6, 8]. In contrast, Botão et al. [8] interviewed 145 individuals from the target population, and 92% said they were willing to receive the vaccine. It is hard to clarify why they showed interest, but the actions were different, but a possible explanation would be that they just manifested agreement for the convenience of the interview or because they fear the authorities. Such attitude toward the government is not new or exclusive to Nampula or northern Mozambique. For instance, Pool et al. [33] reported a similar behavior during a campaign for immunization against malaria 10 years before in Manhiça District, southern Mozambique. Similarly, rumors stated that the local clinic was trying to poison the children. In Gurúè City, people believe that cholera is sent as spells by evil individuals [2]. It would be an asset to investigate what religious leaders or traditional healers think of cholera and government interventions, because it is common for people in Mozambique to rely on them in matters of health, in some cases even for immunization. The fact that conventional practitioners are a direct competition for their source of income cannot be underestimated, and if people, including their leaders and traditional healers, regard outbreaks of diarrhea as a spiritual matter, they might not understand the governments' true motivations, and "conspiracy theories" will keep spreading. Botão et al. [8] reported emerging conflicts related to previous cholera interventions between health professionals, community leaders, and health activists, sometimes escalating to episodes of violence. Interventions seem to become more difficult over time as the locals create barriers for the professionals, and both Botão et al. [8] and Salomão et al. [21] believe only the notion that cholera is life-threatening can motivate the population to accept the vaccine. In any case, prior to vaccination, there should be a strong campaign targeting traditional authorities in order to promote their collaboration and influence the adults, and likewise directed to teachers, to influence the children. It would also include, in the strategy, ways to make sure that people are not absent during the campaigns.

Baltazar et al. [23] also stated that 10% of the individuals experienced side effects after vaccination, and it seems a plausible explanation for the decline of 18.3% in adherence between the two rounds. It is possible that such individuals and their families or relatives preferred not to receive the second dose, and it can still be confirmed if the interview records are available. Minor side effects to this vaccine (Shanchol™) should have been expected in some people [48, 51], and it has been observed in Bangladesh [52]. The vaccination campaign in Nampula was certainly carried with informed consent and following the WHO [53] recommendations, but if the side effects in fact led people to withdraw from the second round, it is important to reevaluate the communication with the target population. The Centers for Disease Control and Prevention [54] recommend competent authorities to explain the people to be vaccinated about the "benefits of and risks from vaccines in language that is culturally sensitive and at an appropriate educational level."

Misdiagnoses should also not be underestimated, especially because it has impact on the choice of treatment. Chissaque et al. [20] reported lack of consistent protocols to directly relate a pathogen with a particular diarrheic profile and also the respective risk factors. Outbreak of a disease can be misleading when there are people carrying diseases with similar symptoms. For instance, Chitio et al. [24] detected *Aeromonas spp.* in 10.4% of 289 samples of rectal swabs from individuals with symptoms consistent with cholera during outbreaks of the latter. Sometimes even conventional culture methods can fail to detect *V. cholerae* [55]. Furthermore, Gupta et al. [56] found that clinical conditions of a coinfection cholera-rotavirus and cholera alone can easily be confused. There should be efforts to ensure rigorous differential diagnoses when it is possible.

Salência et al. [11] reported the abusive use of antibiotics to treat acute diarrhea in children, including confirmed cases of cholera (2.4%), between May 2014 and December 2017 in major hospitals from all regions of Mozambique. According to the authors, antibiotics were used to treat 94% of the patients, and this represents a violation of the WHO's protocol that recommends the use of these compounds when there is cholera, dysentery, and other "recognizable severe cases" [57].

Antibiotic misuse is frequent in developing countries but such level was extreme. For instance, Runesson et al. [58] reported the use of antibiotics in 70% of cases of children with diarrhea, randomly examined in a children's hospital, from which at least 35% did not really need antibiotics. According to Rogawski et al. [59], antibiotics have the potential to modify the gastrointestinal microbiota and increase the risk of a reduced time to a subsequent diarrhea episode. It is also known that antibiotic abuse frequently results in resistance. In 2007, Mandomando et al. [60] reported a high incidence of resistance to chloramphenicol (57.9%), co-trimoxazole (96.6%), and tetracycline (97.3%), and low for quinolone (4.2%). Salência et al. [11] mentioned the use of ampicillin (45%), gentamicin (39%) combined with therapy, and gentamicin (10%). Thus, there should be efforts to discourage physicians to prescribe antibiotics when it is not necessary. When appropriate, they can use quinolone or third-generation cephalosporins [60].

4. Conclusions

The presentations in the XVI National Health Journeys and the recent articles on cholera offered an invaluable contribution to the current knowledge on the disease in Mozambique, particularly regarding the risk factors, health determinants, and immunization process. Such contributions showed how important the journeys were. The Ministry of Health and related institutions have been active in research and interventions to control cholera in Mozambique. The immunization campaign in 2016 certainly had high impact in reducing the incidence of cholera, as no outbreak has been as wide and severe as 2015's (the ones this year are not considered because their extent is still to be assessed). Yet, governmental effort cannot achieve the desired results if there is no collaboration from the civil society. The etiology, risk factors, and epidemiology of the disease are fairly known, and, although the government lacks resources to provide proper sanitation, access to clean water, or vaccine coverage for all people at risk, it is now a matter of designing a strategy to tackle each the issue, and if the plan is solid, funds can be acquired and well used.

5. Recommendations

The following recommendations are not simply observations based on findings shared during the XVI Health Journeys. They are supplemental observations on their actual recommendations, in a broader context if necessary. It seemed unnecessary to bring to light ideas of improvements if the authors have already done so, this being a mere enhancement if they seem incomplete.

Environmental determinants such as water, sanitation, and hygiene synergistically impact the extent of severity of cholera. Thus, Marrufo et al. [4] strongly recommended their evaluation during outbreak-related emergencies. It is true, but such evaluation should not solely occur during outbreaks. Proper management of the way people use water is crucial to prevent outbreaks in the first place, although factors such as heavy rainfall, warm air temperature, or low river flows cannot be controlled, and they increase the exposition of humans to *V. cholerae* [61, 62]. Ramos et al. [19] and Chissaque et al. [20] agreed, but they proposed a more practical approach through construction of specialized improved latrines, adaptable to high levels of the water table, and improved sanitation. Paulo et al. [22] added that it could be done through multi-sectoral groups involving researchers, community leaders, and engineers. It is eventually necessary to act rather than waste plenty of time analyzing the situation, particularly when it urges to make decisions, but

Marrufo's opinion seems more prudent, and it should be the first step, and then the government could consider improvements, still after evaluating their viability. Considering the cost Dengo-Baloi et al. [7] explained the necessity to evaluate how much the Ministry of Health spends for an immunization campaign, but it applies to all forms of intervention and also research. The economic component is crucial, and it should also include how and where to obtain and channel the funds and the best way to manage it in order to prevent unnecessary losses.

Still within the context of health determinants, Borges et al. [5] manifested preoccupations with the people directly using lake water in Niassa, without any treatment, even when they have potable water available. They intended to understand why, and they recommended studies in this direction. They and other authors [6, 22] also think health education campaigns could lead people to understand the risk of such behavior and ultimately take the appropriate measures. The authors are certainly pointing to a constructive direction, but it is a delicate endeavor to convince people to abandon their values and traditions. Niassa Lake, more than a useful water source, is certainly also a source of recreation and economic activities such as fishing or *garimpo*, and the reasons why people use the lake even with water at home might be the same as why urban populations leave their homes to a swimming pool or to the sea for surfing or fishing. Maybe they are moved by the experience, not merely out of necessity. The disbelief in cholera as a bacterial worldwide pandemic in favor of theories of government conspiracy worsens the situation. In this case, particularly if the lake is a source of so many benefits, positive psychology seems to be a more effective direction to consider: showing the benefits of using alternatives (e.g., consuming only treated water) for the same ends rather than repeating how prejudicial the lake water might be. It still means that community education is necessary because people have to know how to prevent cholera.

Chitio and Langa [24] called for a clear definition of cases of *Aeromonas* spp. contaminations during cholera outbreaks to prevent improper treatment. This should not be just for the genus mentioned, but in general physicians should require differential diagnostic for suspected cases of cholera, rather than taking rushed decisions based on arbitrary probability during outbreaks, because it might worsen the problem or create new problems for the patients. If they found that 10% of the cases suspected of cholera were actually related to *Aeromonas* infection, how many might have been related to other causes than *Vibrio* or *Aeromonas*? And which were the consequences of their possible misdiagnosis?

After successfully performing the rapid test for cholera, Dengo-Baloi et al. [18] recommended it as an alternative tool, but they believe that the culture method shall remain to confirm the epidemics, to monitor antibiotic sensitivity, and to produce pure isolates for molecular characterization. Considering how critical outbreaks are, the authors provided a very prudent opinion, and, although their results were highly promising, it is perhaps better to keep testing the method and compare the results with others from authors in different settings before it becomes a standard.

Immunization is already a well-developed area because there are very well-crafted guidelines, based on logical, scientific, and empirical sources, and it has been practiced for many years. Still, healthcare professionals have to face contextual issues, and it results in every-evolving strategies. The door-to-door vaccination strategy seems very effective, and Baltazar et al. [23] said it is better to implement as a preventive measure against potential outbreaks. Having said so, they did not put emphasis on the strategy during outbreaks, possibly because it is preferable to manage the disease when it is easier to control. It is perhaps important to consider the Médecins Sans Frontières [63] recommendations for door-to-door strategies, some of which are already fulfilled. First, it is good that people already have experience with this approach, and there is some acceptance [23]. Second, it is important to coordinate the process with the authorities at neighborhood levels or small communities, where information is easy to spread, and it is also easy to record the number of residents or households in order to keep track of individuals absent during each round and organize catch-up rounds. Baltazar et al. [23] also suggested short-term effectiveness studies, but these have been done and reported by Dengo-Baloi et al. [7] from the same research team. Perhaps the results had not yet been analyzed when Baltazar et al. [23] had already completed their report. To maximize adherence, Botão et al. [8] suggested sensibilization of the population through identification of credible leaders and other influential individualities to function as mobilizers during the entire campaign.

Salência et al. [11] discussed about the indiscriminate use of antibiotic to children with acute diarrhea as a violation of WHO guidelines, and the authors appealed for the optimization of prescription of antibiotics for diarrhea. The authors are correct, but the issue requires perhaps more attention, considering that WHO guidelines result from the international consensus and, in general, physicians are expected to be aware of the dangers of antibiotic overprescription, and this practice is often most likely an act of negligence. Thus, there should be penalties to discourage such kind of misconduct because it is a sensitive public health matter.

The National Health Institute and partners shall keep organizing the National Health Journeys and similar events because they are very constructive platforms in which researchers, scholars, and health professionals can share information and broaden their scope regarding the reality of cholera and other diseases in Mozambique. Such events should be more frequent and organized all over the country to give opportunities to people residing in other areas than the capital city. It would perhaps be a very good idea to promote conferences about the control of cholera or diarrheic diseases in areas of high incidence and engage local health professionals or potential actors who can really influence the current situation.

The final recommendation is based on the words of Chissaque et al. [10] in their summary: the key to control cholera and other diarrheic diseases is a deep understanding of the local epidemiology. Such comprehension would facilitate predictions and planning on how to prevent outbreaks and manage them if they eventually happen. Mozambique could study carefully experiences from other countries where cholera is endemic, such as India or Bangladesh, and understand how they deal with the matter or at least draw some comparisons and interact with foreign scientists. The contexts are surely different, but the problem is similar, and solutions might arise from unexpected variables.

6. Post-conclusive note

There will be soon more updates on cholera in Mozambique because there were two major outbreaks [40, 64, 65], one still ongoing as this manuscript is under preparation [66]. They are related to the intense tropical cyclones Idai and Kenneth that made landfall in Mozambique's central and northern provinces, respectively [67]. According to Miller and Adebayo [37], Kenneth it is the strongest cyclone recorded in the country, and together the tragedies certainly caused the biggest losses since the flood in 2000 [68]. Briefly, Devi [40] said that up to April 20, the Ministry of Health had declared an outbreak due to Idai, and there had been at least 4979 cases of cholera and 6 deaths. Regarding Kenneth, the United Nations Office for the Coordination of Humanitarian Affairs (OCHA) [64] declared that as of 12 May, there were 149 confirmed cases of cholera in Pemba, Metuge, and Mecufi.

Conflict of interest

The authors declare no conflict of interest.

Author details

Edgar Manuel Cambaza[1*], Edson Mongo[1], Elda Anapakala[2], Robina Nhambire[1], Jacinto Singo[1] and Edsone Machava[1]

1 Department of Biological Sciences, Faculty of Sciences, Eduardo Mondlane University, Maputo, Mozambique

2 National Health Institute, Maputo, Mozambique

*Address all correspondence to: accademus@protonmail.com

IntechOpen

© 2020 The Author(s). Licensee IntechOpen. This chapter is distributed under the terms of the Creative Commons Attribution License (http://creativecommons.org/licenses/by/3.0), which permits unrestricted use, distribution, and reproduction in any medium, provided the original work is properly cited.

References

[1] Mesa F, Simbine E, Faranguana AC. Análise de casos de diarreias agudas e óbitos no Hospital Distrital de Mocuba-Junho a Julho de 2015. Revista Moçambicana de Saúde Pública. 2018;**4**:190

[2] Carlos I. Perfil sociodemográfico e cultural dos munícipes da cidade de Gurué, sua relação com a epidemiologia de cólera. Revista Moçambicana de Ciências de Saúde. 2018;**4**:256

[3] Francisco J, Chindia JA. Factores ambientais associados a eclosão e reeclosão da endemia da cólera no Niassa. Revista Moçambicana de Ciências de Saúde. 2018;**4**:134

[4] Marrufo T, Salomão C, Chicumbe S, Muianga C, Cardoso N, Baltazar C, et al. Avaliação de determinantes ambientais (água, saneamento e higiene) na cidade de Nampula em 2016. Revista Moçambicana de Ciências de Saúde. 2018;**4**:66

[5] Borges BV, Armando E, Missage E. Acesso à água, higiene, atitudes e práticas relacionadas com a prevenção da cólera em torno das comunidades do município de Metangula, província de Niassa, 2016. Revista Moçambicana de Ciências de Saúde. 2019;**4**:104

[6] Victorino J, Savaio L, António M. Mitos e boatos da cólera na província de Nampula Janeiro-Março 2018. Revista Moçambicana de Ciências de Saúde. 2018;**4**:149

[7] Dengo-Baloi L, Semá-Baltazar C, Barata A, Malaco C, Chitio J, Muloliwa A, et al. Uso do teste rápido de cólera (modificado) para detectar e monitorar surtos: Monitoria da eficácia da vacina oral contra cólera após campanha de vacinação massiva em Nampula, 2016. Revista Moçambicana de Ciências de Saúde. 2018;**4**:214

[8] Botão C, Paulo J, Chucumbe S, Sinai C, Magaço A, Matsimbe M, et al. Avaliação antropológica: barreiras e facilitadores para aceitação da vacina oral de cólera em Nampula Cidade, 2016. Revista Moçambicana de Ciências de Saúde. 2018;**4**:236

[9] Garrine M, Mandomando I, Vubil D, Nhampossa T, Acacio S, Li S, et al. Minimal genetic change in *Vibrio cholerae* in Mozambique over time: Multilocus variable number tandem repeat analysis and whole genome sequencing. PLoS Neglected Tropical Diseases. 2017;**11**(6):e0005671

[10] Chissaque A, de Deus N, Vubil D, Mandomando I. The epidemiology of diarrhea in children under 5 years of age in Mozambique. Current Tropical Medicine Reports. 2018;**5**(3):115-124

[11] Salência J, Chissaque A, Chilaúle J, Anapakala E, Guimarães E, Manique L, et al. Aderência ao protocolo no uso de antibióticos para tratamento de diarreia aguda em crianças. Revista Moçambicana de Ciências de Saúde. 2018;**4**:86

[12] World Health Organization. The Treatment of Diarrhoea: A Manual for Physicians and Other Senior Health Workers. Geneva, Switzerland: WHO Library; 2005. 44p

[13] World Health Organization, UNICEF. Clinical Management of Acute Diarrhoea: WHO/UNICEF Joint Statement. Geneva, Switzerland: WHO Library; 2004. 8p

[14] Capitine I, Chicumbe S, Chitio J, Langa JP. Avaliação económica da campanha de vacinação com a vacina oral contra cólera em Nampula, Moçambique. Revista Moçambicana de Ciências de Saúde. 2018;**4**:290

[15] Gujral L, Sema C, Rebaudet S, Taibo CLA, Manjate AA, Piarroux R, et al. Cholera epidemiology in Mozambique using national surveillance data. The Journal of Infectious Diseases. 2013;**208**(suppl_1):S107-SS14

[16] Langa JP, Sema C, De Deus N, Colombo MM, Taviani E. Epidemic waves of cholera in the last two decades in Mozambique. Journal of Infection in Developing Countries. 2015;**9**(6):635-641

[17] Vanormelingen K, Le Pechoux M, Bonde T. Cholera Outbreaks in Tete, Sofala, Zambezia, Nampula and Niassa Provinces: UNICEF Mozambique. 2015. Available from: www.unicef.org/appeals/files/UNICEF_Mozambique_SitRep_26_March_2015.pdf

[18] Dengo-Baloi LL, Langa JP, Semá-Baltazar C, Chicumbe S. Avaliação dos eventos adversos pós campanha de vacinação oral contra cólera (EAAI-VOC) em cinco bairros da cidade de Nampula, 2016. Revista Moçambicana de Saúde Pública. 2018;**4**:213

[19] Ramos E, Jasse L, Samo T. A problemática de saúde pública no bairro novo na cidade de Quelimane. Revista Moçambicana de Saúde Pública. 2018;**4**:127

[20] Chissaque A, Deus ND, Vubil D, Mandomando I. Revisão da epidemiologia da diarreia em crianças nos últimos 20 anos em Moçambique (1997-2017). Revista Moçambicana de Ciências de Saúde. 2018;**4**:133

[21] Salomão C, Langa J, Bertil A, Baltazar C. Vacina oral contra cólera, conhecimentos atitudes e práticas, diferenças e igualdades em duas campanhas, Tete 2017-2018. Revista Moçambicana de Ciências de Saúde. 2018;**4**:282

[22] Paulo M, Gurjal L, Cardoso N. Investigação de surto de cólera, na comunidade de Casacone, na província de Nampula, Novembro 2017. Revista Moçambicana de Ciências de Saúde. 2018;**4**:134

[23] Baltazar CS, Baloi LD, Salomão C, Rafael F, Mengel MA, Gessner BD, et al. Cobertura vacinal e aceitabilidade durante a campanha de vacinação contra cólera na cidade de Nampula, 2016. Revista Moçambicana de Ciências de Saúde. 2018;**4**:53

[24] Chitio JJE, Langa JPM. Frequência e perfil de susceptibilidade de *Aeromonas* spp. isolados de surtos de cólera nas regiões centro e norte de Moçambique, 2014-2015. Revista Moçambicana de Ciências de Saúde. 2018;**4**:29

[25] Mocumbi AO. Revista Moçambicana de Ciências de Saúde. Special ed. Maputo, Mozambique: Instituto Nacional de Saúde de Moçambique; 2018

[26] Instituto Nacional da Saúde. Sobre as Jornadas Maputo. 2018. Available from: http://jornadas.insconferencias.co.mz/sobre-as-jornadas/

[27] Domman D, Chowdhury F, Khan AI, Dorman MJ, Mutreja A, Uddin MI, et al. Defining endemic cholera at three levels of spatiotemporal resolution within Bangladesh. Nature Genetics. 2018;**50**(7):951-955

[28] Mutreja A, Kim DW, Thomson NR, Connor T, Hee Lee J, Kariuki S, et al. Evidence for several waves of global transmission in the seventh cholera pandemic. Nature. 2011;**477**:462-465

[29] Hu D, Liu B, Feng L, Ding P, Guo X, Wang M, et al. Origins of the current seventh cholera pandemic. Proceedings of the National Academy of Sciences. 2016;**113**(48):E7730-E77E9

[30] Gradín C, Tarp F. Investigating growing inequality in Mozambique.

South African Journal of Economics. 2019;**87**(2):110-138

[31] World Health Organization, United Nations Children's Fund. Drinking Water | JMP: World Health Organization (WHO) and United Nations Children's Fund (UNICEF). 2019. Available from: https://washdata.org/monitoring/drinking-water

[32] Seibert G. "But the Manifestation of the Spirit Is Given to every Man to Profit Withal": Zion Churches in Mozambique since the Early 20th Century. Le Fait Missionnaire. 2005;**17**:125-150

[33] Pool R, Munguambe K, Macete E, Aide P, Juma G, Alonso P, et al. Community response to intermittent preventive treatment delivered to infants (IPTi) through the EPI system in Manhica, Mozambique. Tropical Medicine & International Health. 2006;**11**(11):1670-1678

[34] World Health Organization. WHO | Areas Affected by Cholera Epidemics: World Health Organization. 2016. Available from: https://www.who.int/gho/epidemic_diseases/cholera/epidemics_text/en/ [Updated: 26 September 2016]

[35] Ansaruzzaman M, Bhuiyan NA, Safa A, Sultana M, McUamule A, Mondlane C, et al. Genetic diversity of El Tor strains of *Vibrio cholerae* O1 with hybrid traits isolated from Bangladesh and Mozambique. International Journal of Medical Microbiology. 2007;**297**(6):443-449

[36] Wikimedia Commons. File: Mozambique sat.png. San Francisco, California, USA: The Wikimedia Foundation Inc. 2006. Available from: https://en.wikipedia.org/wiki/File:Mozambique_sat.png

[37] Miller B, Adebayo B. Cyclone Kenneth. Thousands Evacuated as Mozambique is hit with the Strongest Storm in its History. Atlanta, Georgia, USA: Cable News Network. 2019. Available from: https://edition.cnn.com/2019/04/25/africa/cyclone-kenneth-mozambique-evacuation-intl/index.html

[38] World Health Organization. WHO | Cholera Case Fatality Rate: World Health Organization. 2017. Available from: https://www.who.int/gho/epidemic_diseases/cholera/case_fatality_rate_text/en/ [Updated: 18 September 2017]

[39] Schnoering K. Mozambique Cyclone Idai Response. UN Migration; 2019. Report No.: 2

[40] Devi S. Cyclone Idai: 1 month later, devastation persists. Lancet (London, England). 2019;**393**(10181):1585

[41] Anjichi-Kodumbe T, Abreu S, van Vliet T. Southern Africa: Tropical Cyclone Kenneth Flash Update No. 8: United Nations Office for the Coordination of Humanitarian Affairs (OCHA). 2019. Available from: https://reliefweb.int/sites/reliefweb.int/files/resources/ROSEA_20190503_SouthernAfrica_TCKenneth_FlashUpdate8_DRAFT.pdf

[42] Anjichi-Kodumbe T, Abreu S, van Vliet T. Southern Africa: Tropical Cyclone Kenneth Flash Update No. 7: United Nations Office for the Coordination of Humanitarian Affairs (OCHA). 2019. Available from: https://reliefweb.int/sites/reliefweb.int/files/resources/ROSEA_20190501_SouthernAfrica_TCKenneth_FlashUpdate7_FINAL.pdf

[43] Cabral D, Balde T, Schmachtel C. Tropical Cyclone Idai, Mozambique: Donor Alert. Geneva, Switzerland: World Health Organization; 2019

[44] Chingwaru W. Letters to the Editor: How to Keep Cholera and Typhoid at Bay in the Post Cyclone Idai Period:

@ChronicleZim. 2019. Available from: https://www.chronicle.co.zw/letters-to-the-editor-how-to-keep-cholera-and-typhoid-at-bay-in-the-post-cyclone-idai-period/

[45] Jeuland M, Lucas M, Clemens J, Whittington D. A cost–benefit analysis of cholera vaccination programs in Beira, Mozambique. The World Bank Economic Review. 2009;**23**(2):235-267

[46] George CM, Rashid MU, Sack DA, Bradley Sack R, Saif-Ur-Rahman KM, Azman AS, et al. Evaluation of enrichment method for the detection of *Vibrio cholerae* O1 using a rapid dipstick test in Bangladesh. Tropical Medicine & International Health. 2014;**19**(3):301-307

[47] Ontweka LN, Deng LO, Rauzier J, Debes AK, Tadesse F, Parker LA, et al. Cholera rapid test with enrichment step has diagnostic performance equivalent to culture. PLoS One. 2016;**11**(12):e0168257

[48] Shantha. Cholera Vaccine (Inactivated, Oral) I.P. Shanchol Mahape, Navi Mumbai, India: Sanofi Pasteur India Private Limited. 2014. Available from: https://www.stopcholera.org/sites/cholera/files/shanchol_insert_3-2015.pdf

[49] Khan IA, Saha A, Chowdhury F, Khan AI, Uddin MJ, Begum YA, et al. Coverage and cost of a large oral cholera vaccination program in a high-risk cholera endemic urban population in Dhaka, Bangladesh. Vaccine. 2013;**31**(51):6058-6064

[50] Khan AI, Levin A, Chao DL, DeRoeck D, Dimitrov DT, Khan JAM, et al. The impact and cost-effectiveness of controlling cholera through the use of oral cholera vaccines in urban Bangladesh: A disease modeling and economic analysis. PLoS Neglected Tropical Diseases. 2018;**12**(10):e0006652

[51] World Health Organization. Use of Oral Cholera Vaccine in Humanitarian Emergencies. Geneva, Switzerland: World Health Organization; 2014. Available from: https://www.who.int/cholera/vaccines/OCV_in_humanitarian_emergencies_15Jan2014.pdf

[52] Saha A, Chowdhury MI, Khanam F, Bhuiyan MS, Chowdhury F, Khan AI, et al. Safety and immunogenicity study of a killed bivalent (O1 and O139) whole-cell oral cholera vaccine Shanchol, in Bangladeshi adults and children as young as 1 year of age. Vaccine. 2011;**29**(46):8285-8292

[53] World Health Organization. WHO Recommendations for Routine Immunization—Summary Tables. Geneva, Switzerland: World Health Organization; 2019. Available from: https://www.who.int/immunization/policy/immunization_tables/en/

[54] Centers for Disease Control and Prevention. Preventing and Managing Adverse Reactions. Atlanta, Georgia, United States: Centers for Disease Control and Prevention; 2017

[55] Alam M, Hasan NA, Sultana M, Nair GB, Sadique A, Faruque AS, et al. Diagnostic limitations to accurate diagnosis of cholera. Journal of Clinical Microbiology. 2010;**48**(11):3918-3922

[56] Gupta S, Jhamb U, Uppal B, Chakraverti A, Mittal SK. Diagnosing cholera in the young: A review of WHO criteria. JK Science. 2007;**9**(3):137-139

[57] Bruzzese E, Giannattasio A, Guarino A. Antibiotic treatment of acute gastroenteritis in children. F1000Res. 2018;7:193

[58] Runesson J, Shamansurova E, Jacobsson G. Antibiotics are being misused to treat diarrhoeal disease in children in Central Asia. Acta Paediatrica (Oslo, Norway: 1992). 2016;**105**(12):1382-1383

[59] Rogawski ET, Westreich DJ, Becker-Dreps S, Adair LS, Sandler RS, Sarkar R, et al. Antibiotic treatment of diarrhoea is associated with decreased time to the next diarrhoea episode among young children in Vellore, India. International Journal of Epidemiology. 2015;**44**(3):978-987

[60] Mandomando I, Espasa M, Valles X, Sacarlal J, Sigauque B, Ruiz J, et al. Antimicrobial resistance of *Vibrio cholerae* O1 serotype Ogawa isolated in Manhica District Hospital, Southern Mozambique. The Journal of Antimicrobial Chemotherapy. 2007;**60**(3):662-664

[61] Jutla A, Whitcombe E, Hasan N, Haley B, Akanda A, Huq A, et al. Environmental factors influencing epidemic cholera. The American Journal of Tropical Medicine and Hygiene. 2013;**89**(3):597-607

[62] Camacho A, Bouhenia M, Alyusfi R, Alkohlani A, Naji MAM, de Radiguès X, et al. Cholera epidemic in Yemen, 2016-2018: An analysis of surveillance data. The Lancet Global Health. 2018;**6**(6):e680-e690

[63] Médecins Sans Frontières. Chapter 4: Strategies for epidemic response. 2018 [cited 7 June 2019]. In: Management of a Cholera Epidemic: Practical Guide for Doctors, Nurses, Laboratory Technicians, Medical Auxiliaries, Water and Sanitation Specialists and Logisticians [Internet]. Geneva, Switzerland: Médecins Sans Frontières; 7 June 2019. Available from: https://medicalguidelines.msf.org/viewport/CHOL/english/4-7-vaccination-strategies-23448968.html#

[64] Anjichi-Kodumbe T, Abreu S, van Vliet T. Southern Africa: Tropical Cyclone Kenneth Flash Update No. 13: United Nations Office for the Coordination of Humanitarian Affairs (OCHA). 2019. Available from: https://reliefweb.int/report/mozambique/southern-africa-tropical-cyclone-kenneth-flash-update-no-13-12-may-2019

[65] Isbell T, Bhoojedhur S. Cyclones add to Mozambique's Public Health Challenges. 2019. Available from: https://www.afrobarometer.org/publications/ad297-cyclones-add-mozambiques-public-health-challenges

[66] United Nations Office for the Coordination of Humanitarian Affairs. Southern Africa: Tropical Cyclone Kenneth: United Nations Office for the Coordination of Humanitarian Affairs (OCHA). 2019. Available from: https://reliefweb.int/report/mozambique/southern-africa-tropical-cyclone-kenneth-flash-update-no-8-3-may-2019

[67] Isbell T, Bhoojedhur S. Cyclones add to Mozambique's Public Health Challenges/Ciclones aumentam os desafios de saúde pública em Moçambique South Africa: Centre for International Governance Innovation, South African Institute of International Affairs. 2019. Available from: https://www.africaportal.org/publications/cyclones-add-mozambiques-public-health-challenges-ciclones-aumentam-os-desafios-de-sa%C3%BAde-p%C3%BAblica-em-mo%C3%A7ambique/

[68] Filipe J. In: Muiambo P, editor. Moçambique 2000: As Águas da Morte. 1st ed. Maputo: Moçambique Editora Lda.; 2003. 191p

Section 4

Status of Mental Health in Older Adults: Treatment and Prevention

Chapter 10

Exploring Mental Health Treatment and Prevention among Homeless Older Adults

Ramona Bullock-Johnson and Karen Bullock

Abstract

Homelessness is an issue of social justice, in the United States, because it leaves people vulnerable, unsafe, and ill, while not having their basic needs for food and shelter met. Although the United States is the wealthiest country in the world, a significant number of its residence, whether citizens or not, have experienced homelessness in their lifetime. Less than 5 years ago, the U.S. Department of Housing and Urban Development (HUD) found that 564,708 people are homeless on any given night. There is a dearth of information available that puts older adults at the forefront or at the center of homelessness epidemic. Moreover, recent HUD reports claim that homelessness has decreased, in the United States, while the National Center on Family Homelessness reported that the number of residents experiencing homelessness is steadily climbing and is expected to hit an historic high, within the next 5 years. Yet, most of the attention given to homelessness as a public health issues, tends to focus on families and children. Few studies have targeted older adults and their primary risk factors experiencing homelessness. Important to note is the fact that consistent data and accurate reporting about homeless older adults are few and far between. This chapter (1) presents a practical definition of homelessness, (2) provides a social work framework for understanding and assessing risk among homeless populations, as well as, (3) emphasizes the importance of cultural competence in health practices for addressing homelessness among older adults as a public health concern.

Keywords: older adults, mental health, homelessness

1. Introduction

The United States, the population is aging, and increasingly more adults are aging into poverty. At the same time, housing is becoming more unaffordable and the costs of health care are rising, leaving older adults at risk of poverty and homelessness [1]. Healthcare access for older adults is an important public health issue to be addressed globally. In the United States, approximately 10,000 people turn age 65 daily, and as the population ages in general, the prevalence of homeless among older adults remain constant [2]. Based on recent demographic trends, the more than 44,000 older adult population accounted for in 2010 will more than double by the year 2050, to nearly 93,000 [3].

Much is written in the health promotion literature about the social determinants of health for older adults, generally and more specifically, as it relates to disease and health promotion [4]. Moreover, it is well documented that a range of personal, social, economic, and environmental factors contribute to individual and population health [5, 6]. Specifically, people with better education, more stable employment, stable housing and living arrangements, and access to preventive health services tend to be healthier across the life course [7, 8]. Conversely, poor health care outcomes are often made worse by a lack of access and opportunities to engage in health social and physical environments [9, 10].

Worth noting is a surveys of patients' experiences with health care services that revealed how well a country's health system can be observed as meeting the needs of its population. Using data from a 2016 survey conducted in 11 countries—Australia, Canada, France, Germany, the Netherlands, New Zealand, Norway, Sweden, Switzerland, the United Kingdom, and the United States—research found that adults living in the United States (U.S.) reported poor health and well-being and were the most likely to experience accessibility hardships. Furthermore, the U.S. lagged behind other countries in making health care affordable and ranked poorly on providing timely access to medical care. Deficits in patient engagement and chronic care management were reported, in all countries, and at least one in five adults experienced a care coordination issue or problem. In particular, often, such challenges had high levels of acuity for low-income adults. In the Netherlands, performance at the top of the 11-country range on most measures of access, engagement, and coordination was noteworthy as models of best practices [8].

From a psychological and legal perspective, researchers in the United States have argued that access to mental healthcare for diverse public health populations need improvement, if progress is to be made in the areas of addiction and recovery [11]. Sixty percent of people with mental illness do not get the mental healthcare that they need, and up to 90% of those with a substance abuse disorder do not receive services [12]. Some of the hindrances to those who need to receive mental healthcare include the negative stigma surrounding mental illness, cost of care, limited access in rural areas, and lack of transition between services, among other things. These obstacles have an even greater impact on those in the population without insurance, or lacking sufficient mental health coverage, and those who cannot afford to pay out of pocket for these services. Individuals within some minority groups often do not have the same health resources as the majority [13]. Adding these facts to the number of mentally ill people within the homeless population, it appears that those who need the services the most may be unable to obtain it.

The history of homelessness, from a policy standpoint indicates certain patterns of viewing the issue of homelessness, and paints a picture of why the public perception is focused on the individual person and not the structure of our society. Current policies intended to address homelessness can be improved with the incorporation of social work frameworks and perspectives on creating more equitable, social and distributive justice treatments and interventions [14], as well as, affordable healthcare, public and political opinions span the necessary action or inaction of dealing with the social problems at the patient, provider, and policy levels, especially mental health services. Unfortunately, many fail to recognize the need for healthcare for the aging population. According to the World Health Organization [6], 15% of adults aged 60 and over suffer from a mental disorder. There are several mental disorders that older adults may be diagnosed with; including dementia, depression, anxiety disorder, or substance use problems. According to the American Psychiatric Association [15], one in four older adults experience some type of mental disorder. This number is expected to rise over the next several years due to the overall increase among the aging population.

Certain characteristics indicate the hypocrisy within mainstream U.S. society's view of the homeless, specifically the homeless that are veterans [16, 17]. In spite of the fact that the prevalence of homelessness is paramount and has many contributing factors, less humane approaches are taken to help them gain self-efficacy to be well, emotionally and spiritually. According to National Coalition for the Homeless [18], single individuals comprised 66.7% of all people experiencing homelessness (369,081 people), and about 33.3% are people in families (184,661 adults and children). Based on these data, approximately 7.2% are older adults and according to the National Coalition for the Homeless, some argue the number negatively impacted is too small to give an abundance of attention and resources. This marginalization of older adults should not be tolerated nor condoned. Especially, in the United States (US) which is often viewed as the "land of opportunity" or the "home of the free and the brave." Yet there are many people living in this country that do not have the means for basic human necessities like food and shelter, and older adults are disproportionately impacted [14, 42]. The perception of life in the US, in the general public, is far different than the reality of increasingly more people who have little to no "opportunity" and some segments of the population feel they are neither "free nor brave" enough fight to against the inequities and discriminatory practices that oppress them on a daily basis. In struggling to deal with this overwhelming adversity, there is often no attention or time made for the self-care of homeless individuals with substance use disorders (SUD).

From a Social Work perspective, what is understood about the standard of practice is the importance of looking for resources and strategies for assisting marginalized, disenfranchised, poor and underserved individuals, families, groups, communities, and a host of others. The Social Work Code of Ethics [19] speaks to the value of social justice, as well as, social and political action. To advocate for health care reform and especially, for the most effective intervention approaches, so that people can have greater access to mental health and substance abuse intervention is in keeping with the Code for the profession of social work.

Older adults, consistent with the reports on younger and middle-aged adults are impacted by substance use and addiction in ways that are shaped by biological, psychological, and social factors [11]. The social learning theory (SLT) suggests that homelessness, as well as, addiction recovery models are rooted the very opinions and beliefs that are perpetuated and learn from years of social conditioning and exclusion of specific racial and ethnic minority cultural preferences, norms and attitudes toward healthcare. Treatments based on this theory can disrupt patterns of negative thought and patterns of maladaptive behavior.

Racial disparities in treating mental health disorders are widely discussed in the healthcare literature [16, 20–23]. Yet, differences in use of recommended strategies to prevent homelessness as a mental health intervention, by race/ethnicity, have not been widely examined. Racial disparity in homelessness among older adults to growing national concern and questions about barriers to service provision, with little attention given to association between health literacy and mental health care; especially trauma-informed care. Once of few studies was conducted to examine the impact of diversity attributes on health care literacy, and this end, statistical data analysis on a nationally representative sample of 15,309 respondents was published [24]. The study revealed a significant difference between ethnic/racial minorities, as well as, between men and women. Most notable were the differences between social, economic, and educational factors that influenced outcomes. This research is especially relevant to the topic of older adults, race/ethnicity and effective prevention and intervention of homelessness. Furthermore, national advocacy reports and federal government sponsored initiatives consistently document the health disparities that racial and ethnic minority persons experience [23, 42].

More specifically, racial minority groups, in the U.S., experience disproportionately higher rates of homelessness, than racially White groups. In considering homelessness as a public health problem that requires attention to access and acceptability of healthcare, food, shelter and social support, the clear link for older adults is the strong correlation between mental health and homelessness [11].

2. Homelessness, mental health and substance use disorders

A practical definition of substance use is one of the most commonly described and identified health risks among people experiencing homelessness [25]. Homelessness is defined as the absence of a permanent home. Individuals and families may live on the streets, in a shelter, a single room occupancy facility, abandoned building or vehicle, or in any other unstable or non-permanent living arrangement (Section 330 of the Public Health Service Act (42U.S.C., 254b)). For more than a decade, studies reporting on the experiences of homeless persons have examined the association between living arrangement and substance use disorder treatment program characteristics, because housing instability is known to impact mental health and SUD prevention and intervention efforts [17, 26]. Substance use among older adults, specifically who are homeless, is associated with decreased mobility of physical and mental health capacity [25] and early onset morbidity and mortality [27]. For these reasons, more attention on older adults as a special population of concerns for mental health prevention and intervention is warranted.

3. Approaches and frameworks

Behavioral modification interventions have been proven to be effective. These approaches are client-centered and provide support for abstinence from substance use. Moreover, such flexible models of care offer a range of modifiable frameworks for addressing attitudes and behaviors related to addiction and recovery [28]. In the field of social work practice, in particular, problem-solving frameworks are often recommended because of the evidence-based, culturally informed, manualized strategic tools that give mental health care provider the options to tailor the intervention to diverse populations and can be implemented in a range of different settings, including clinics, hospital, community-based environments and even in-home services with older adults, specifically [22, 29].

Arguably, mental health intervention should take more of a community-based prevention approach versus a medical model, institutional treatment, when tailored to, and for persons living in homeliness [11]. The debate about the degree to which homeless persons will be able to access services to address their problems of substance use disorders, as well as, home and food insecurity, rest squarely on macro-level factors, including policies, legislation, research for evidence-based recommendations and solutions. The World Health Organization (WHO) recognizes mental disorders a public health concern, worldwide and its use of the term "disorder," implies the existence of observable behaviors or symptoms that interfere with normal functioning and that cause distress. Homelessness can exacerbate the symptoms of mental illness, causing an individual to become debilitated, depressed and anxious, all of which can be costly, socially and economically for individuals and families. Prevention of mental disorders and effective interventions, as well as, population-based policies that support and foster health accessibility among all person, are among the ongoing challenges that countries, worldwide must contend with [30]. In the U.S., culturally specific approaches to addressing mental health prevention and intervention among older adults is an important aspect of health care access.

4. Promising preventive strategies using a cultural competence framework

A cultural competence framework is one that guides healthcare providers' behaviors, attitudes, value and perspective on caring for individuals, families and communities. The culturally competent service provider takes into account an individual's multiple identities, preferences, norms, beliefs, as well as, their social determinants of health. The way in which healthcare providers' social and professional experiences impact their worldview, particularly as it relates to their delivery of care to diverse populations and it influences how and to what degree they are willing to ensure equity and parity in the mental healthcare services they provide. Furthermore, while homelessness is not considered to be a determinant of mental illness, interdisciplinary research and evidence-based theories suggest a strong correlation race culture, homelessness and access to healthcare [12, 13, 31]. Mental health providers have argued that it is extremely challenging to implement standard intervention strategies with this diverse population. The stigma associated with aging and mental health can make it rather difficult for providers to understand how to facilitate the same approaches with housing secure individuals, as one would implement with older adults living with homelessness. Changing the views and perspectives require a cultural competence lens through which to see and experience prevention and intervention this older adult populations. Based a comprehensive literature review, self-care and mindfulness are useful supporting cognitive behavioral modification interventions with person's managing mental health and substance use disorders [14]. These strategies may well have lasting, positive impacts on health outcomes. Promising preventive strategies for addressing mental health care among older persons that are homeless require a range of varied interventions. Some additional recommended approaches include self-help groups, integration of spiritual/religious beliefs, reminiscence therapy that incorporates the focus of balanced review and reflection of one's past life, and/or interdisciplinary clinical pharmacological treatments, as needed to maintain activities of daily living, physical exercise, and psychosocial health, while in recovery from substance use and homelessness [32]. The adaptation to cultural norms, attitudes and preference can increase accessibility and acceptability [13, 17, 22].

Cognitive behavioral literacy therapy using books, audiotapes, and video presentations also has been shown to alleviate mild depressive symptoms through promotion of self-help [33]. Such audio and video media for the elderly should take into consider educational level, readability, font size, and use of examples relevant different cultural groups. For example, appropriate content targeting older adults transitioning out of homelessness could involve retirement planning that includes development of positive expectations of a new life phase, a change of environment, developing new interests and stronger social support networks.

Preventive strategies aimed specifically at elders' spiritual/religious beliefs have been shown to be more effective than treatment-as-usual which neglects such beliefs and related practices [34]. These strategies may include religious participation involving prayer, spiritual music consumption, emotional and psychological preparation for an afterlife, a review of one's life journeys, and/or spiritual counseling. Research has shown [35] that involvement in spiritual/religious activities led to decreased depression among some other adults. In the U.S., the 12-Step model of addiction recovery has principles that guide the processes [36] and one of the core components is 'belief in a higher power.'

Reminiscence or life review therapy has yielded mixed results [33]. This potentially preventive approach involves literally reviewing one's life experiences as far back as one can remember and examining each life stage in terms of one's choices and the consequences of those choices for self and others. Given that the consequences of such experiences could be either positive or negative, perhaps it is the attitude toward such consequences that is critical to the effectiveness of this approach for prevention. If one believes that life is an opportunity to learn, then the results of the life review may prove to be positive and instructive for further learning and avoiding the same mistakes, thereby allowing for self-correcting and a sense of perceived control.

Psychodynamic therapy has also been evaluated empirically continue to have popularity as an approach within a managed care environment that reimburses only empirically supported treatments for older adults [33]. With homeless older adults, such interventions have been facilitated in substance abuse recovery program and in other shelter-based program that address mental health conditions, including SUDs [11].

Pharmacotherapy may also be an effective prevention strategy with older adults and there are a number of recommendation for addressing risk and side effects of antidepressant medication when prescribed to older adults, and especially those that are in addiction recovery [37]. One precaution is that approximately 20% of older adults have serious health problems that can be aggravated by antidepressant medications, including increased risk of physical injuries and hypertension disorders [33]. Moreover, research suggests that anti-anxiety and other sedative medications worsen conditions of depression and perhaps anxiety, among older people with substance use disorders [38–42]. Noteworthy is caveat methodological flaws and limitations may contribute to these negative findings in the research. Variations in interventions techniques, provider characteristic and sociocultural diversity of the participants are not clearly explained and such omissions can result in ambiguous and confounding effects.

5. Summary

As a moral imperative, fundamental in the profession of social work, the core value and belief that every human being deserves a home, food, clothing and access to health care compel us to make this call to action. Older adults should not be excluded from the inalienable rights and dignities, worldwide [19] to have their basic needs met. As the risk of homelessness among older adults increases, this becomes a public health and human right concern for healthcare systems and providers. This call to action for expedient problem-solving to prevent older adults from living in poverty and becoming homeless. Solutions are within our local, regional, national and global reach, such as expanding and strengthening the existing safety net of health care and minimum income supports, such as Temporary Assistance for Needy Families (TANF), Child Support Enforcement, Medicare and Medicaid, as well as, including a livable wage for those whom continue to be employed. An increase in the supply and accessibility of affordable housing for the aging population and low-cost or no-cost community based mental health and substance disorder prevention and intervention services are a few of the recommended solutions [42].

Author details

Ramona Bullock-Johnson and Karen Bullock*
North Carolina State University, Raleigh, NC, USA

*Address all correspondence to: kbulloc2@ncsu.edu

IntechOpen

© 2020 The Author(s). Licensee IntechOpen. This chapter is distributed under the terms of the Creative Commons Attribution License (http://creativecommons.org/licenses/by/3.0), which permits unrestricted use, distribution, and reproduction in any medium, provided the original work is properly cited.

References

[1] The Henry J. Kaiser Family Foundation. Poverty Among Seniors: An Updated Analysis of National and State Level Poverty Rates Under the Official and Supplemental Poverty Measures. 2015. Retrieved form: http://files.kff.org/attachment/issue-briefpoverty-among-seniors-an-updated-analysis-of-national-and-statelevel-poverty-rates-under-the-official-and-supplemental-povertymeasures [Retrieved: 15 June 2019]

[2] Justice in Aging. How to Prevent and end Homelessness among Older Adults. Special Report. 2016. Retrieved from: https://www.justiceinaging.org/wp-content/uploads/2016/04/Homelessness-Older-Adults.pdf

[3] Sermons MW, Henry M. Homelessness Research Institute. The Demographics of Homelessness Series: The Rising Elderly Population. 2010. Retrieved from: http://www.endhomelessness.org/files/2698_file_Aging_Report.pdf [Retrieved: 15 June 2019]

[4] Office of Disease Prevention and Health Promotion. Social Determinants. 2015. Retrieved from: https://www.healthypeople.gov/2020/leading-health-indicators/2020-lhi-topics/Social-Determinants/determinants [Retrieved: 1 July 2019]

[5] Gatz M, Smyer MA. The mental health system and older adults in the 1990s. American Psychologist. 1992;**47**(6):741-751. DOI: 10.1037/0003-066X.47.6.741

[6] World Health Organization. Ageing and Health. 2017. Retrieved from: https://www.who.int/news-room/fact-sheets/detail/ageing-and-health [Retrieved: 23 June 2019]

[7] Hudson CG, Chafets J. A comparison of acute psychiatric care under Medicaid carve-outs, HMOs, and fee for service. Social Work in Public Health. 2010;**25**(6):527-549

[8] Osborn R, Squires D, Doty M, Sarnak D, Schneider E. In new survey of eleven countries, U.S. adults still struggle with access to and affordability of health care. Health Affairs. 2016;**35**(12):2327-2336. DOI: 10.1377/hlthaff.2016.1088

[9] Ball S, Bullock K. Retirement satisfaction. In: Gullota T, Bloom M, editors. Encyclopedia of Primary Prevention and Health Promotion. 2nd ed. Vol. 4. New York, NY: Springer Publishers; 2014. pp. 2095-2105

[10] Lee CM, Mangurian C, Tieu L, Ponath C, Guzman D, Kushel M. Childhood adversities associated with poor adult mental health outcomes in older homeless adults: Results from the HOPE HOME Study. American Journal of Geriatric Psychiatry. 2017;**25**(2):107-117. DOI: 10.1016/j.jagp.2016.07.019

[11] Fitzpatrick DC, Hall JK, Bullock K. Addiction and long-term recovery among diverse homeless populations. In: Maschi T, Leibowitz G, editors. Forensic Social Work: Psychological and Legal Issues with Diverse Populations and Settings. New York, NY: Springer Publishing; 2017. pp. 293-304

[12] Cummings JR, Lucas SM, Druss BG. Addressing public stigma and disparities among persons with mental illness: The role of federal policy. American Journal of Public Health. 2013;**103**(5):781-785. DOI: 10.2105/AJPH.2013.301224

[13] Saloner B, Le Cook B. Blacks and Hispanics are less likely than Whites to complete addiction treatment, largely due to socioeconomic factors. Health Affairs. 2013;**32**(1):135-145

[14] Bullock-Johnson R. Homelessness and Substance Use Disorders: The Need for Self-Care and Mindfulness. NASW Mental Health Specialty Practice Section News Magazine. Washington, DC: National Association of Social Worker; 2019

[15] American Psychiatric Association. DSM-5, Diagnostic and Statistical Manual of Mental Disorders. 5th Revised ed. Washington, D.C.: American Psychiatric Association; 2013

[16] Tsai J, Mares A, Rosenheck R. Do homeless veterans have the same needs and outcomes as non-veterans? Military Medicine. 2012;**177**(1):27-31

[17] Zerger S. Substance Abuse Treatment: What Works for Homeless People? A Review of the Literature. 2002. Retrieved from: http://www.nhchc.org/wp-content/uploads/2011/09/SubstanceAbuseTreatmentLitReview.pdf

[18] National Coalition for the Homeless. Mental Illness and Homelessness. 2017. Retrieved from: http://nationalhomeless.org/wp-content/uploads/2017/06/Mental-Illness-and-Homelessness.pdf [Retrieved: 24 March 2019]

[19] National Association of Social Workers. Code of Ethics of the National Association of Social Workers. Washington, DC; 2017

[20] American Psychological Association. Mental Health Disparities Among Racial and Ethnic Minorities: What Providers Should Know. 2019. Retrieved from: https://www.apa.org/pi/disability/resources/mental-health-disparities [Retrieved: 3 June,2019]

[21] Buka SL. Disparities in health status and substance use: Ethnicity and socioeconomic factors. Public Health Reports. 2002;**117**(Suppl 1):S118-S125

[22] Bullock K, Allison H. Access to medical treatment for African American populations: The current evidence base. In: Christ G, Messner C, Behar L, editors. Handbook of Oncology Social Work. New York, NY: Oxford University Press; 2015. pp. 293-298

[23] Substance Abuse and Mental Health Services Administration. Racial/Ethnic Differences in Mental Health Service Use among Adults. Rockville, MD: U.S. Department of Health and Human Services Publication; 2015. Publication No. SMA-15-4906

[24] Rikard RV, Hall JK, Bullock K. Health literary as a barrier to trauma-informed care across diverse groups. Traumatology. 2015;**21**(3):227-236

[25] Substance Abuse and Mental Health Services Administration. Results from the 2013 National Survey on Drug Use and Health: Summary of National Findings. 2013. Retrieved from: https://www.samhsa.gov/data/sites/default/files/NSDUHresultsPDFWHTML2013/Web/NSDUHresults2013.pdf [Retrieved: 27 May 2019]

[26] Guerrro EG, Song A, Henwood B, Kong Y, Kim T. Response to culturally competent drug treatment among homeless person with different living arrangements. Evaluation and Program Planning. 2018;**66**:63-69

[27] Zivanociv R, Milloy MJ, Hayashi K, Dong H, Sutherland C, Kerr T, et al. Impact of unstable housing on all-cause mortality among persons who inject drugs. BMC Public Health. 2015;**15**:106. DOI: 10.1186/s12889-015-1479-x

[28] Amodeo M, Lundgren I, Cohen A, Rose D, Chassler D, Beltrame C, et al. Barriers to implementing evidence-based practices in addiction treatment programs: Comparing staff reports on motivational interviewing, adolescent community reinforcement approach, assertive community treatment, and cognitive-behavioral therapy.

Evaluation and Program Planning. 2011;**33**(4):382-389

[29] Helfrich CA, Chan DV, Sabol P. Cognitive predictors of life skill intervention outcomes for adults with mental illness at risk for homelessness. American Journal of Occupational Therapy. 2011;**65**:277-286. DOI: 10.5014/ajot.2011.001321

[30] World Health Organization. Prevention of Mental Disorders: Effective Interventions and Policy Options. Summary Report. Geneva, Switzerland: World Health Organization; 2015. pp. 1-65. Retrieved from www.who.int/mental_health/evidence/en/prevention_of_mental_disorders_sr.pdf

[31] Drake RE, O'Neal EL, Wallach MA. A systematic review of psychosocial research on psychosocial interventions for people with co-occurring severe mental and substance use disorders. Journal of Substance Abuse Treatment. 2011;**34**(1):123-138

[32] Gary RA, Dunbar SB, Higgins MK, Musselman DL, Smith A. Combined exercise and cognitive behavioral therapy improves outcomes in patients with heart failure. Journal of Psychosomatic Research. 2010;**69**:119-131

[33] Karel MJ, Hinrichsen G. Treatment of depression in late life: Psychotherapeutic interventions. Clinical Psychology Review. 2000;**20**:707-729

[34] Monod S, Rochat E, Büla C, Spencer B. The spiritual needs model: Spirituality assessment in the geriatric hospital setting. Journal of Religion, Spirituality, & Aging. 2010;**22**:271-282

[35] Levin J. God, Faith, and Health: Exploring the Spirituality-Healing Connection. New York: John Wiley & Sons, Inc.; 2001

[36] National Institutes of Health. National Institute of Drug Abuse—Principles of Drug Addiction Treatment: A research Based Guide, 3rd ed. 2018. Retrieved from: https://www.drugabuse.gov/publications/principles-drug-addiction-treatment-research-based-guide-third-edition/frequently-asked-questions/are-there-specific-drug-addiction-treatments [Retrieved: 10 June 2019]

[37] Guay DRP. Geriatric pharmacotherapy updates. The American Journal of Geriatric Pharmacotherapy. 2010;**8**:86-96

[38] Whitaker R. Anatomy of an Epidemic: Magic Bullets, Psychiatric Drugs, and the Astonishing Rise of Mental Illness in America. New York: Crown Pub; 2010

[39] Hall JK, Bullock K. A practicum partnership approach to addressing barriers to mental health among racially diverse older adults. International Journal of Humanities and Social Science. 2015;**5**(8):10-19

[40] Jansson BS. The Reluctant Welfare State: Engaging History to Advance Social Work Practice in Contemporary Society. 7th ed. Belmont, CA: Brooks/Cole Publishers; 2012

[41] Kessler RC, Berglund P, Demler O, Jin R, Merikangas KR, Walters EE. Lifetime prevalence and age-of-onset distributions of DSM-IV disorders in the National Comorbidity Survey Replication. Archives of General Psychiatry. 2009;**62**:593-602

[42] National Alliance to End Homelessness. Changes in the HUD Definition of "Homeless." 2012. Available from: https://endhomelessness.org/resource/changes-in-the-hud-definition-of-homeless/